ABOUT THE AUTHOR

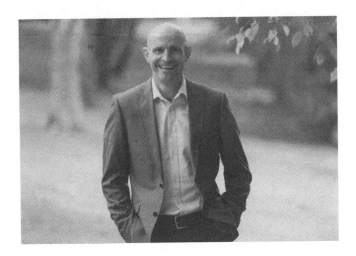

Mark Bunn is a former professional Australian Rules (AFL) footballer, uniquely trained in both Western and ancient Eastern health sciences.

Specializing in Ayurvedic medicine (Maharishi Ayurveda) he has also extensively researched the lives and secrets of the world's healthiest and longest living people.

A featured health and wellbeing expert in the International Best-Selling 'Millionaire Book Series', Mark has also authored a number of online health programs. One of Australasia's most booked conference speakers, he presents his inspiring, uplifting seminars in multiple countries each year on mind-body health, happiness, life balance, meditation, spirituality and consciousness.

Mark is also a trained teacher of Transcendental Meditation (TM), and supports the David Lynch Foundation for disadvantaged youth and war veterans and the Beyond Blue national depression initiative.

markbunn.com.au
facebook.com/Mark.Bunn.EasternWisdom
linkedin.com/in/markbunn

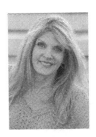

"The ancient wisdoms of that Mark speaks and writes about are absolutely fascinating and life changing. I love Ayurveda and Mark is one of the precious few people in the world who can explain its wisdom so practically for use in our modern lives. Highly recommend!"

Kathy Smith—New York Times best-selling author with a revolutionary approach to fitness, inspiring millions of people to lose weight and adopt a healthier lifestyle—www.kathysmith.com

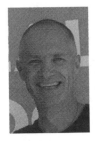

"... this book has been by far the best-selling book we have stocked, outselling books such as 'The Power of Now' by Eckhart Tolle, and Patrick Holford's 'Optimum Nutrition Bible.' It's been just phenomenal. A guy just came back and bought 30 more copies for all his friends and family."

Jason Gunn—Founder of Oliver's Real Food Stores—Sydney, Australia

What Others Are Saying About
'Ancient Wisdom for Modern Health'

"Finally a book written with exactitude and simplicity in its unveiling of much needed longevity and Ayurvedic secrets. As a life long seeker of truth, a 35 year daily practitioner of yoga and meditation, and a 15 year yoga teacher, I joyfully recommend this book to all my students and my self-improvement peers."
Richard Esquinas—The American Yogi, Japa Yoga founder & official "yogi of record" for The Arnold Classic (Governor Arnold Schwarzenegger).

"If you want to get to the core of what it takes to be really, really healthy with tons of vitality and positive energy, and achieve this naturally, then read this book from cover to cover."
Raamon Newman—Managing Partner, Raam Global Partners—Los Angeles, USA

"... enjoyable, easy to read, and packed full of useful and easy to apply tips that you can apply to your daily life. Many Ayurvedic books are very complex and not very user friendly, but this book unravels this comprehensive system and makes it practical for everyone."
Vicki Broome—Leading Ayurvedic Practitioner—Johannesburg, South Africa

This beautiful and incredibly helpful book is one of the few books I've ever read that has actually helped me to easily and specifically improve my health physically, mentally and even spiritually. It feels like a loving friend who is there by your side, inspiring you toward your healthiest and best self!
Karen Kondazian—International & USA award-winning author of "The Whip"

"A really terrific book for helping people to re-enliven the simple truths of health and to remember how simple health and happiness should be."
Paul Mendlesohn—CEO of CODE—United Kingdom

"... straight-forward advice from science with meaningful mindfulness from the east. It's a marriage of ideals that really works for optimal health, vitality and true work-life balance. I love this book."
Dr Joanna McMillan—Channel 9's (Today Show) Nutritionist & Practising Dietitian

"In the modern era, many people have lost their peace. Mark Bunn, who has extensively studied ancient scriptures and teachings, reminds us of the age-old wisdom of our own Ayurvedic tradition and Ayurvedic masters, for returning to a more peaceful and meaningful life. If you want to achieve a 'happier' as well as a 'healthier' life, this book will enlighten your path."
Rajendra Kher—5 time Award-winning Indian author

"Great book! Health & wellness for mind, body and soul. Not only makes sense, but is so simple. I wish I knew all of this years ago!"
Matt Welsh—World champion & world record holding swimmer

"I am a Spanish personal trainer who absolutely loved your book! Ever since I read it, I have tried to stick to the seven wisdoms. Your way of bringing smiles and laughs all the time is just fantastic. You could also be a comedian! I will also say that since I read your book my family and I squat when we go to the toilet and...by God!...it is so much easier! Lol!"
Elsa Ciria—Madrid, Spain

"No nonsense, common sense information ... free of fads and gimmicks ... that delivers on its promise and contains excellent examples of simple, timeless wisdom for better health & happiness."
Catherine DeVrye—Former Australian Executive Woman of the Year & Best-Selling Author

"Mark. Thank you very much for your book—a copy is in our library and many doctors have already read it. I have just come from giving some lectures in Uttar Kashi and your book helped me a lot. Many patients and doctors will read it. Again, thank you very much."
Dr Jagabandhu Nath—Senior Doctor at Khosla Medical Institute (Maharishi Ayurveda Hospital)—Delhi, India

ANCIENT WISDOM

for
Modern Health

Book One
The Essential Wisdoms

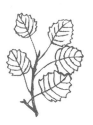

rediscover the simple, timeless secrets
of health and happiness

Mark Bunn

Cataloging-In Publication entry:

Bunn, Mark.
Ancient Wisdom for Modern Health: Book One–'The Essential Wisdoms'

6th Edition (2017)
Includes references and index.

ISBN 978-0-9807597-0-9 (pbk.)

Bunn, Mark. Ancient Wisdom for Modern Health series; Book 1.

Health. Happiness. Mind-body. Medicine, Ayurvedic.

158.1

Published by Enlightened Health Publishing (Mark Bunn)
E-mail: info@markbunn.com.au

10% of the profits of this book go to supporting the
Beyond Blue national depression initiative and the David Lynch Foundation
www.davidlynchfoundation.org

To the now late but great Karen,

*for your constant support, wise input, and most
importantly, for the many times you
re-inspired me to continue on with this book.
In whatever form you are, I will love you always.*

Contents

A life-changing discovery

Health and happiness ...
were never meant to be complicated

Nature's way is simple and easy,
but men prefer what is intricate and artificial.
Lao Tzu

Do you get frustrated when every week there seems to be another book, magazine article, TV show or groundbreaking research study saying the exact opposite of what you were told the week before? Dairy is good. No, dairy is bad. Red meat increases your risk of cancer and heart disease. No, red meat is essential for optimal health. Short duration, high intensity exercise is best ... er, sorry ...!

Just a few short years after finishing a degree in Western health science, I too was frustrated and confused. Having spent years studying the latest scientific information on fats, calories, vitamins, free radicals, anti-oxidants and aerobic training zones, I was struggling to keep up. One month it was a 'revolutionary new' weight loss diet, the next it was another 'scientifically proven' exercise program, and the next it was the latest 'miracle supplement' for impotence. Besides the fact that few of the diets and none of the supplements actually worked (er, so I was told!), it was all so complicated.

Then, in early 1994, I had one of those moments when in an instant your life is changed forever. I was given a book on Maharishi Ayurveda, a modern-day restoration of the ancient system of Ayurvedic medicine. I read about how health and wellbeing were not meant to be complicated at all. Eating was not about calories, fats and waistlines. It was about enjoyment, communal connection and nourishing the body's inner intelligence. Exercise was not about optimal heart rates, having a six-pack or looking good in a bikini. It was about unifying mind, body and soul, and for promoting higher states of consciousness.

As soon as my football career finished, I travelled to south-east Asia. I loved going out into remote villages and seeing how the people lived, often as their families had done for centuries. I was fascinated by their simple way of living. However, what struck me most about these 'simple folk' was that while most of them barely possessed a roof over their heads and the clothes on their backs, they were nearly always smiling and laughing and seemed genuinely happy. Furthermore, apart from problems relating to nutritional deficiencies (due to their restricted diets) and poor sanitation, they were also generally robust, strong and hardy. All this was despite their distinct lack of material possessions, challenging life circumstances and limited access to modern medicines. The greatest irony hit me when I returned home to Australia. I saw people everywhere with relative riches and supposedly the best health system in the world, yet drowning in depression, anxiety, stress, obesity and a myriad of other health conditions. We certainly didn't seem to be as happy or contented as the supposedly less civilized, 'backward' people I had just visited.

Intrigued by such a dichotomy, I began to research the ancient Eastern traditions of health care. At the time, all I knew of the Eastern world was how good they were at producing world-class leg spinners and curries that could burn holes in your underpants! Little did I know that they possessed thousands of years of the most profound health wisdom. It was then that the next lightning bolt struck me. I learnt that in contrast to the Western understanding, from the Eastern perspective, ill health and chronic disease were seen to be more a result of violating certain fundamental laws of life than an inevitable part of aging. Our bodies were understood to possess their own in-built wisdom, and if we lived in ways that enlivened that wisdom or intelligence, good health was the natural result.

I felt blessed to have the opportunity to complete formal studies in Maharishi Ayurveda, and then to witness this knowledge in practice. Travelling around Australia for almost two years with an international team of doctors trained in this approach, I got to sit in on hundreds of personal consultations. Patients would come in with chronic conditions that had been plaguing them for weeks, months, even years. Time after time, with often nothing more than changes to their diet, daily routine and lifestyles (many of which are outlined in the pages to come), they experienced profound improvements in their symptoms. Many shed excess kilograms they had not been able to budge in years. Some began sleeping again after months of insomnia. Others experienced significant relief from—or even overcame—long-standing medical conditions. Nearly all regained lost energy and enjoyed a renewed zest for life.

Fascinated by the idea that good health was actually our natural state, I began researching the healthiest and longest-living peoples of our time. I was astounded to find that even today, there are cultures living right under our noses where a large percentage of individuals live exception-ally long lives, experiencing few of the physical or mental diseases that are widespread in the Western world. Throughout all my studies, what became most apparent was that there were certain basic principles of health (health wisdoms) common to nearly all long-surviving indigenous cultures, time-tested natural health sciences and the age-old Eastern tra-ditions of knowledge. Individuals and cultures throughout time that have tended to enjoy relatively happy, disease-free lives have more often than not followed these universal, timeless truths. It is these people that I consider to be among the world's healthiest. They may not all have lived 'long' lives necessarily, but they have predominantly lived happy, purposeful lives in harmony with the world around them.

As previous authors have already more than adequately outlined many of the individual habits common to healthy, long-living individuals, in this book I have attempted to focus more on the basic principles or wisdoms that underlie health, happiness and long life. I have tried to complement these wisdoms where appropriate with recent modern scientific research. I have done this in the hope that the suggestions given will have maximum practicality for you within a busy Western lifestyle.

Some quick notes to help your reading

i) Ancient wisdom

The basis of the knowledge discussed in this book comes from what could be called the collective wisdom of human experience. You will often hear me refer to general terms such as 'ancient wisdom', 'natural wisdom' or 'wise teachers throughout time' as the foundation of points made. While specific examples will also be cited on occasion, these terms are used to signify the collective wisdom that has been gained and maintained by many of our forebears throughout time. This includes knowledge from time-tested natural health sciences, the practices of long-living individuals, as well as the teachings of enlightened spiritual men and women. Rather than citing numerous examples each time, the point is that common understandings of the essential keys to healthy living are universal. Whether from Indian yogic masters, Tibetan holy men, Chinese or African medicine men, wise Aboriginal or Native American elders, intuitive healers of the South Americas, or any number of other sources, the real wisdoms of health and happiness are timeless and unchanging.

ii) Ayurveda

Although there are many cultures and traditions throughout the world that have understood and preserved a rich knowledge of life and health, in this book I will often draw on the knowledge contained in the science of Ayurveda. Ayurveda dates back over 6000 years and is widely considered the world's oldest continuous system of health care. Ayurveda literally means 'science of life' and is based on the universal, eternal laws of nature that have governed our world since the dawn of time. As such, its basic teachings are applicable to all people, in all places, at all times. While my training was specifically in Maharishi Ayurveda, as this is a very precise body of knowledge recently re-enlivened by far more enlightened minds than mine, I do not make any attempt to try and represent this profound knowledge here. Instead, I have simply tried to keep to basic principles and have used the general terms of 'Ayurveda' or 'Ayurvedic medicine'. However, if you are interested in the general Ayurvedic principles touched on in this book, I can highly recommend further investigation into this wonderful approach. (Some further background information regarding these topics can be found in the ebook that accompanies this book. Details about the ebook are outlined in the box at the end of this chapter.)

iii) Simple wisdoms ... but not necessarily easy

As you will soon discover, most of the wisdoms contained in this book are nothing other than simple truths you already know—if not consciously then at least intuitively. While they are simple to understand, however, I am the first to admit that many of the wisdoms are not always easy to implement. I certainly don't pretend to be able to follow them at all times and know it can be difficult for others.

Just a few years ago, someone very close to me was diagnosed with a serious health condition. It was, and in some ways still is, one of the most difficult times of my life. It certainly gives me immense compassion for you, should you or someone close to you be going through some form of sickness or ill health. Even now, with the greatest motivation to stay connected to the simple wisdoms of health, I admit that I find it extremely challenging at times to do everything I know is healthy. Modern life doesn't always make it easy. If you have a hectic working life or are a mother or father with two or three young children, I can only imagine how difficult certain things may be for you. However, while the practicalities may be challenging, if we truly desire better health and greater happiness in life, at some point making changes in the direction of the principles of health is arguably the most 'practical' thing we can do.

It always intrigues me that we can see it as practical to spend $50,000 on heart bypass surgery and live permanently on cholesterol lowering medication, but it's not practical to change our diet. It's not practical to change jobs so that we can have a less stressful life and get more exercise, but it's okay to be chronically overweight and subject ourselves to life-threatening diabetes. It's not practical to meditate or go and get some fresh air and sunshine, but it's practical to be constantly tired, regularly stressed or to live with chronic (though avoidable) illnesses. Maybe the most practical thing we can do individually and collectively is to start reconnecting to the age-old wisdoms of health.

I invite you to join the growing wave of people reverting back to the simple, natural ways of health, and hope that within this book you may remind yourself of one or two nuggets of our ancestral wisdom that will help you live a long and happy life. I wish you the very best of health.

Mark Bunn

Supplementary ebook:

To help you get maximum value from this book, an accompanying ebook has been produced.

It contains a number of additional resources, suggestions and further information to help you implement some of the ideas presented. Before you proceed, feel free to obtain your complimentary copy by going to markbunn.com.au/awmh1_ebook

Part I

The wisdom of wisdoms

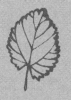

Live in Harmony with Mother Nature's Laws

Health and beauty are gifts of nature
for those who live according to her laws.
Leonardo Da Vinci

Imagine that underlying our material universe, there was a secret code that clearly spelled out all of its mysteries.

Imagine that we could all enjoy vibrant health and happiness if we simply had access to that code. Like modern-day scientists who are searching for the secret genetic code to uncover the mysteries of why we get certain diseases, many cultures throughout history—the ancient Greeks, Chinese, Indians, Peruvians, Mayans and various Native American tribes—have known that there is a set of laws that clearly and precisely explains every detail of our world. Of course, these laws are not really meant to be a secret at all. They are not mysteriously hidden or lost in some ancient tomb or ruin, waiting for Indiana Jones to rediscover them. The real secret is that the basic keys to living a long and healthy life are not contained in a concrete, physical form at all. They do not lie outside of us. They lie within us and within our connection to the natural world.

In recent times, in our quest to uncover the secrets to life and health, we have progressively distanced ourselves from the natural world. As a result, many of the traditional wisdoms that guided the health and progress of civilizations before us have become lost beneath a mountain of (often confusing) scientific facts and figures. In many indigenous cultures, secret wisdoms of life have been passed down in oral traditions since time immemorial. The Aborigines still understand the primordial patterns and seed wisdoms of our world through the knowledge of their Dreamtime. The American Indians, through their dances and stories, maintain a deep connection to the eternal 'spirit that moves through all things'. The ancient hymns of India are not simply religious prayers, they are a preserved record of the sacred sounds that underlie all of life and contain 'the knowledge by which all other knowledge is known'.

Fortunately, in many instances these wisdoms have also been recorded in written form to serve as a guiding light for people to maintain health in harmony with the natural world. For almost every 'revolutionary' breakthrough in modern science, there are a dozen traditional cultures that have known how to prevent the corresponding condition for thousands of years. Recent scientific 'discoveries' that certain herbs can have powerful medicinal effects—like ginger in combating nausea, cinnamon in decreasing blood sugars, and turmeric in breaking down brain plaques—have all been recorded in traditional medicine systems for centuries.

Analyze less ... live longer!

Esmerelda Stavra lived on the Greek island of Symi. She was 107 when she died. Her son and daughter-in-law, Manoles and Maria, said: 'Her house was at the top of the village steps, and even when she was 100 years old she went up and down them three or four times a day so that she could sell the feta cheese and yoghurt she made'. Esmerelda was never sick during her lifetime and never went to a check-up with the doctor. Maria added, 'When she died, my mother thought she had just gone to sleep—that's how quietly she went'.[1]

Not a bad sort of life, is it? Sure beats having a chronic illness for much of your life and spending your last years isolated in a nursing home in varying degrees of pain and discomfort. The story of Esmeralda Stavra appears in Sally Beare's pioneering book 'The Live Longer Diet'. In it, Beare gives an exceptional account of a number of the world's longevity hotspots—places where a high percentage of individuals live to well beyond the average life span. In discussing Symi, she says, 'Right up to their nineties, men and women can be found chasing after their herds, collecting herbs, making yoghurt and gardening'. Campodimele, in southern Italy, is known as Europe's 'village of eternal youth'. Beare comments, 'It is rare for anyone to die before the age of 85, and Campodimelani often reach their nineties and even sail past 100 without ever having to visit the doctor'.[2]

Although we spend trillions (yes, trillions) of dollars each year searching for new miracle drugs or genetic-based panaceas to help combat the myriad diseases that plague us, there are many people throughout our world who have lived to ripe old ages with almost a complete absence of such diseases. In his wonderful book 'Healthy at 100', John Robbins writes about how, in the early 1970's, Professor Alexander Leaf went on behalf of National Geographic magazine to study some of the longest living peoples of the world. These included the Hunzans of remote Pakistan, the Abkhasians of the Caucasus regions of southern Russia, and people from the Ecuadorian valley of Vilcabamba.[3]

What did he find?

Not only was a high percentage of people living to 80, 90 and 100 plus years of age, many still maintained high levels of physical activity, good mental acuity, healthy blood pressures, low cholesterol, strong bones, a great sense of humor, and a general zest for life. While most suffered the typical hardships of life and their lives were not perfect by any means, they still managed to enjoy predominantly vibrant, happy lives with minimal physical or mental deterioration. Many lived until old age without 'growing old'.

Many similar cultures, tribes and communities also exist through-out the world. Until recently, cancer, heart disease, diabetes, osteoporosis and Alzheimer's disease, amongst other diseases, have been almost unheard of in certain parts of rural China, on the famous Japanese island of Okinawa and in certain Native American cultures. What is most fascinating, however, is how much these cultures have known about the latest and greatest revelations from the world of science.

> The majority of the healthiest, longest living individuals throughout history have never heard the results of even one scientific study on health.
>
> They have never heard of good fats, bad fats or low carbohydrate diets, and would screw up their faces in ignorant pain if you started talking about omega 3's, anti-oxidants, phytochemicals, glycaemic index, good bacteria or optimal heart rates.
>
> We Westerners almost drown in such information—yet have rates of cancer, heart disease, diabetes, obesity and stress disorders in epic proportions.[a]
>
> Do you think we might be missing something?
>
> So what is the secret to these people's health and longevity?

Although genetics is undoubtedly a factor, it does not seem to be the major one. When healthy individuals from traditional cultures migrate to Western countries and take on Western diets and lifestyles, they generally begin to suffer the same type and degree of our diseases within a short space of time. 'The China Study' is a best-selling book based on the world's most comprehensive study on nutrition ever conducted.[4] In it, T. Colin Campbell details the results of a survey of death rates from cancer of more than 880 million citizens of China, of whom 96% were of

---

a   Although in the West we are living longer than ever before, in most cases the onset of serious disease—obesity, diabetes, heart disease—is occurring at younger and younger ages. Thus, while modern technology is allowing us to delay dying, most people are simply extending the number of years they are living with chronic diseases. That is, we are not necessarily living longer, we are just 'dying' longer.

a Chinese ethnic background. The study resulted in a color-coded atlas of cancer rates throughout China. Despite the genetic backgrounds being similar from place to place (87% of the population at that time were from the same ethnic group, the Han people), huge variations in cancer rates were seen. In close to a billion Chinese at least, the clear indication was that cancer was largely due to environmental or lifestyle factors, not genetics. Campbell also cites the authors of a major review on diet and cancer prepared for the US Congress in 1981, which estimated that genetics only determines about 2-3% of the total cancer risk.[5] Many other studies show that while there are certain genetic predispositions to common Western diseases, it is environmental and lifestyle influences such as nutrition that are most important in determining whether we activate or turn on these genes.

A number of other factors have also been put forward to explain the health and longevity of such groups. These include the high fish consumption of the Okinawans, the vigorous daily exercise performed by the Hunzans, the attitude of pragmatic realism commonly found among centenarians on the Italian island of Sardinia, and the abundance of fresh air, clean water and natural foods common to other long-living populations. While such practices would no doubt contribute a favorable influence on health and aging, it is unlikely that any individual behavior in isolation would account for such dramatic differences in health outcomes. What seems evident is that those who have tended to enjoy good health and a relatively long life have consciously or unconsciously lived in tune with some deeper, collective principles of life. To appreciate what this might entail and to isolate one underlying factor common to health and longevity, we need to dig a little deeper. We need to look to the underlying laws of life.

The timeless recipe for good health—follow Mother Nature's laws

Sickness is the vengeance of nature for the violation of her laws.

Charles Simmons

Just as we have man-made societal laws—'thou shalt not kill' or 'thou shalt not steal'—which are designed to promote order and progress in society, the ancient Ayurvedic sages declared that there are a number of natural laws that promote order, progress and evolution in our world.

Think of the world we live in. Our seasons come at certain times and in a certain sequence every year. Winter follows summer. Day follows night. Birds migrate, penguins march, and bears hibernate according to some unseen but guiding intelligence that promotes their health and survival. Being intimately connected with the natural world around us, there are also specific laws that we humans are subjected to. Electro-magnetism, the boiling point of water and the ebb and flow of the tides are all examples of universal laws that express the precise, intelligent functioning of nature and give order and predictability to how we live.

Importantly, just as there are natural laws that govern the rhythms and flow of life generally, there are certain laws of nature that govern the rhythms and flow of our individual bodies. Basic 'natural laws' govern everything from our digestion, our elimination, our hormones, our sleep cycles, our brain functioning, our emotions through to our internal healing mechanisms. When we live in harmony with these laws, rather than violating them as we commonly do in modern Western society, all our physiological functions attract the support of Mother Nature. Like swimming downstream instead of upstream, everything flows better, maintaining good health becomes simpler, and we experience more ease in life. When we truly understand these laws, we can have as much confidence in knowing what foods, exercise, vocations and relationships are best for us as we have in knowing that the 'law' of gravity will make the apple from the apple tree fall to the ground.

Age-old principles of natural health

Though there is an infinite number of natural laws, underlying these are some general principles of health. These principles have formed the basis of the most successful traditional health sciences and the more advanced cultures throughout time. It is good to remind ourselves of these basic understandings as they form the foundation of all health and healing.

1. Our universe has an underlying intelligence.

There is an order and innate harmony underlying everything in nature. At the basis of our physical world is a non-physical intelligence. We can see the expression of this unseen intelligence in everything from the workings of our solar system, the changing of the seasons to the growth of a newborn child.

2. We are intimately connected to this intelligence—our bodies are by nature 'intelligent'.

As understood by all long-surviving indigenous cultures, we are not separate from the world around us. The intelligence that runs our universe is the same intelligence that runs our bodies. Fundamental to maintaining good health and wellbeing is promoting and supporting our body's inner intelligence by aligning it with the cycles and rhythms of the natural world. As we will see, this includes practices such as minimizing the intake of food after the sun sets and rising early in the morning with the sun.

3. Our bodies are self-renewing and self-healing—given the right ingredients.

Rather than being concrete physical machines, doomed to decay, deterioration and disease, our bodies, being inherently intelligent, have a tremendous capacity to repair, rebuild and renew themselves. We see this in everything from overcoming a cold or repairing a bruise to mending broken bones. If given the right basic ingredients to support the body's natural self-healing mechanisms, they can also do this with respect to more serious conditions such as heart disease, diabetes and even cancer. These basic ingredients, or 'natural medicines', are what comprise Part II of this book ('The seven wisdoms').

4. Health is our natural state.

Combining all of this understanding, the ultimate reality is that our bodies are exquisitely built for health. Experiencing good energy, vitality and wellbeing is the natural state of life when we live in accord with the natural laws of life. We do, however, have free choice. By violating or moving away from the basic principles of health, ill health can arise.

5. Our own inner wisdom is our ultimate guide.

Ultimately, our bodies guide us to what we need for balance through our subtle intuitions and gut feelings. Though we commonly fail to listen to or dismiss these inner messages in favor of expert opinions or the latest scientific findings, they represent our body's supreme healing wisdom. Whether feelings of pain or unease, a desire for more rest, a craving for certain foods, or an inkling that something is not quite right, our bodies are always giving us feedback. When we stop and listen to these internal guides, we access our body's highest wisdom.

> If we were to isolate one factor common to the world's healthiest and longest living populations, it would be that they have predominantly lived in harmony with the natural laws of life.
>
> By living in tune with Mother Nature's laws, we take advantage of her almighty intelligence, strength and power. Good health flows more naturally, we don't age as quickly, and we experience greater joy in life.
>
> Like a surfer riding the waves of the ocean, Mother Nature does all the work and we simply enjoy the ride.

Seed wisdom

In solely looking for the secrets to health and longevity under microscopes or inside petri dishes, we have lost sight of many of the essential wisdoms of our ancestors. In constantly searching outside ourselves, we have forgotten that the true secrets to health and happiness lie within.

Part II

The seven wisdoms

Wisdom One

Nourish the Heart Before Nourishing the Body

*You cannot fall in love and
catch a cold at the same time.*[1]

Who is healthier: the person who eats the perfect diet but hates their job and is constantly critical of themselves—or the person whose diet is at best average but loves what they do and feels contented with their lot in life? Who is more likely to die young: the person who exercises for two hours a day and has a washboard stomach but lives in a toxic relationship—or someone who is a few kilos overweight but is happily married, laughs often and enjoys the loving support of friends and family?

While it would be unwise to diminish the benefits of eating well or being fit, if we were to ask the enlightened sages of times past, or even many modern-day neuroscientists, the latter examples would more likely be suggested as the healthiest in the true sense of the word. The reason is that while diet and exercise are vitally important, the ancients knew that the unseen, non-physical world of our emotions affects our health most profoundly. The Swnwt or 'Lady Doctors' of ancient Egypt, based everything they did in the art of healing on their understanding that 'health comes from a happy heart.'[2] These words were also inscribed at the top of the Pharaohs' tombs in Giza. Even back then it was understood that, to a large degree, our emotions create our physical reality. Modern science too is now starting to confirm this wisdom.

'Broken heart syndrome' is a relatively new medical term. It is used to describe individuals who have experienced severe emotional stress, such as the breakup of a relationship or the death of a loved one, and as a result develop heart attack-like symptoms. If you have ever had your heart broken, you might remember how painful this can be physically. *'White coat hypertension'* is another well-known medical term used to explain how people's blood pressure increases just before they are to see their doctor. (Apparently rectal prostate examinations in men cause the most pronounced increases!)

In a study based on over 2 million deaths from natural causes, Dr David P. Phillips of the University of California found that women were more likely to die in the week after their birthdays, while men tended to die shortly before their birthdays. The most likely cause for the difference is purported to be that women correlate birthdays emotionally with friends, family and celebration, so look forward to them. However, men often associate birthdays with things like re-assessing goals, seeing if they have achieved targets and meeting *dead*lines. Such events, where there is an increase in distress around the anniversary of an event, are now known as *'anniversary reactions.'*

In all these cases—broken heart syndrome, white coat hypertension and anniversary reactions—nothing physical happens, yet the most concrete and tangible physical changes occur. All such examples, of which there are thousands more, confirm that how we feel on the inside is even more important than what happens to us on the outside.

According to ancient Eastern wisdom and the natural laws of life, physical medicines come a long way down the list in comparison to medicines of the heart.

Better to be happy than have a perfect diet. Better to be happy than be supremely fit.

Happy thoughts = happy body

Many people today would dismiss the idea that it is better to be happy than have a healthy lifestyle. That's because, until recently, Western science has largely dismissed the powerful effects of our abstract feelings and emotions. However, the wisest teachers throughout time have taught us that our unseen thoughts have far-reaching physical effects. Jesus said, 'As you think so shall you be'. And Buddha, 'All that we are is a result of what we have thought'. Natural health sciences such as Ayurveda suggest that our inner world of feelings and emotions has even more profound effects on our physical health than our day-to-day thoughts. This is because the emotional or *feeling mind*' as it is sometimes called is known to operate at an even deeper level of our human machinery than our thinking mind.

The following diagram illustrates this.

GROSSEST LEVEL

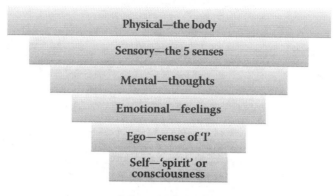

Physical—the body

Sensory—the 5 senses

Mental—thoughts

Emotional—feelings

Ego—sense of 'I'

Self—'spirit' or consciousness

SUBTLEST LEVEL

Diagram 1: Experiences (positive or negative) on the emotional level spontaneously create related effects on the grosser levels of our mind (thoughts), senses and body. This is because our feelings operate on a more fundamental level of our being than our everyday thoughts. As the ancients foretold, our hearts are both electrically and magnetically stronger than our brains. More powerful than our mental thoughts are the emotions deep in our hearts.

Just as radio waves are unable to be seen, yet travel throughout space and time creating tangible, concrete effects (like music), the latest discoveries of mind-body medicine show how our thoughts and feelings do the same. Neourotransmitters, or brain chemicals in layman's speak, have been shown to have receptors on immune system cells throughout our entire body.[3] What this suggests is that whatever is going on in our mind is communicated to our immune system. Receptors for pain-reducing opiates exist not only in our brain but in our stomach and intestines.[4] Today's research demonstrates that the cells of our body are literally chatting to each other every second of the day.[5] Every idea, nuance of thought, whim or feeling we have is gossiped to every other cell in our body through the language of chemistry, electricity and vibrational energy in the blink of an eye. Indeed, ancient spiritual masters have suggested that our dominant feelings not only change the chemical and electro-magnetic fields within us but also *around us*. This may explain phenomena like auras, the so-called subtle 'emotional energy bodies' and even how we can feel uplifted, peaceful or uncomfortable just by being around certain people.

Essentially, we help create the internal environment in which we live, and quite likely our nearby external environment, through the thoughts in our heads and the feelings in our hearts. Even more importantly, science is beginning to detail how different emotions each have their own unique molecular or biological signature. The internal chemistry and thus the effects of love, happiness and joy are distinctly different from the emotions of sadness, stress or anger. Literally, happy feelings create happy molecules. Anxious feelings create anxious molecules. In a similar way, the ancient Eastern sciences also understood that each different emotional state has its own distinct vibrational frequency. Experiencing love and joy produces a vastly different cellular vibration than feelings of worry or guilt. Whether coming from an ancient or modern perspective, the consensus is the same. The happier we feel, the happier our cells are. The happier our cells are, the more harmoniously and intelligently they function, and the more likely they are to keep us healthy.

> Happy thoughts = happy body.
> Stressed thoughts = stressed body.
> Sexy thoughts ...... we wish! Lol!

Feeling good—medicine par excellence

Many years ago, a Georgetown University study showed that our physical and emotional hearts are interconnected. When participants were emotionally stressed, the ability of their hearts to fill with and pump blood was greatly compromised. When we think of health conditions such as angina (heart pain), stroke and heart disease, we usually associate them with physical factors such as high cholesterol and high blood pressure. However, many studies now demonstrate even stronger connections between these diseases and non-physical events. In men, these influences include how fulfilled they are in their work, how happy they are in life generally and even whether they feel loved at home.[6] One particular study done in 2004, involving a 23-year follow-up of over 10,000 middle-aged Israeli men, showed they had a higher risk of dying from stroke when there were perceived family difficulties or when they felt that their wife and children tended not to listen to them.[7]

The good news is that it is not just negative emotions that affect our health. Positive emotions do too. Three decades ago, researchers at Ohio State University were studying atherosclerosis—the build-up of plaque in the arteries. They inadvertently found that the cholesterol levels of rabbits were reduced by up to 60% when they were stroked and petted for a few minutes before being fed a high cholesterol diet (as compared to rabbits who were fed like ordinary lab animals). 60%! If a pharmaceutical company developed a new pill that could naturally reduce cholesterol by 60% without any side effects, it would be front page news across the world. Patients would be banging down doctors' doors and the company would be rolling in billion dollar profits. Yet simply reducing stress and taking more time to be affectionate or intimate with our loved ones may very well deliver similar results. I can just see the National Heart Foundation recommending that we should 'lovingly stroke a friend or partner before eating dinner'! Maybe they should. It would sure be a lot cheaper (and safer) than the billions of dollars spent each year on cholesterol lowering drugs.

In more recent times, a 2010 study published in Europe's leading cardiology journal suggested that experiencing positive emotions may help prevent heart disease. Over a period of ten years, 1,739 healthy men and women were assessed for what's known as 'positive affect'—the experience of pleasurable emotions such as joy, happiness, excitement, enthusiasm and contentment. Researchers found that people with no positive affect were at a 44% higher risk of heart attack or angina than those with a moderate positive affect.[8]

A lot is said about the French and Italian cultures having relatively low levels of heart disease, despite fairly rich, high fat diets. Common explanations point to the anti-oxidants in the wine they consume, the prevalence of olive oil in their cuisine, and the freshness of their food. The fact that they don't scoffit all down in two bites followed by a couple of slugs of coke would certainly help too. However, what is often overlooked is the emotional connection. Some years ago a sociological study was performed where people from France and America were each shown a piece of rich chocolate cake. They were asked what first came into their mind on seeing the cake. The overwhelming consensus of the French was that of pleasure, joy and 'celebration'. Almost unanimously, the Americans' overriding emotion was that of... 'guilt'!

In contrast to cultures such as the French and Italians, in our culture, food and eating is often connected with guilt, coping with emotional stress, or counting points for the latest diet plan. Have you ever seen women on diet plans eating cheese and crackers while sipping a glass of wine? Most of them don't even enjoy it because they are so focused on how many 'points' they are accumulating. It's almost as if they are eating and drinking points rather than something to be enjoyed and savored. At McDonald's, they always ask, 'Do you want fries with that?' But wherever we eat, it could well be asked, 'Would you like pleasure or guilt with that?' and then, 'Do you want low-fat, standard or double guilt?' The reason all this is important is that it's not just fats and calories that our bodies need to metabolize, it is also the biochemical residues of whether we feel guilty or joyous when we eat.

> In time, factors such as our emotional state will be found to be the most critical influences on how we metabolize our food. This is because feeling good and being happy literally change the biological pathways by which we process, absorb and assimilate food.

The ancient Vedic sages knew all about the power of our emotional state. That's why for thousands of years before 'modern science', the timeless Ayurvedic texts have encouraged people to eat only when settled and happy. Eating when anxious or upset was known to disturb the internal digestive processes, such that even the healthiest food could literally become poison to the body. There is little in the way of modern scientific research in this area. However, most of us have experienced eating a large meal of rich foods while laughing and joking with friends and family in a relaxed, jovial atmosphere. At the end of the night we feel full but satisfied. We lean back, pat our bellies and say 'Ah, that was good'. The next night, we eat the exact same food alone in front of the evening news (this alone is usually enough to throw anyone's digestion out), and we feel so bloated and heavy that we can't get off the couch. The reality is, how we feel when we eat is just as important as what we eat. Better to be happy and eat a slightly less than perfect diet, than to have the perfect diet but eat without joy.

In Ayurveda, the experience of enjoyment and pleasure is not only considered of primary importance in terms of diet but in everything from exercise to conception. In former times, to aid conception, the first prescription for any prospective father and close family members was to make the intended mother-to-be happy. While extensive recommendations about what foods, herbal preparations and even sexual practices to promote conception were also known, in the ancient texts it is said, *'a happy woman can conceive at any time'.* It is understood that when a woman is happy and contented on the deepest level, the subtle channels responsible for the proper nourishment and transportation of reproductive materials 'open like a lotus'. This allows the all-important life energy to flow unimpeded, and promotes the optimal environment for fertility. It is interesting to note the experiences of many couples who endure years of anguish trying to conceive, often involving many attempts at procedures such as IVF. If unsuccessful, they eventually resign themselves to the fact they will probably never have children. Though understandably heart-wrenching, it can sometimes also be a significant emotional relief. When they finally give up and stop trying, it is not uncommon for them to fall pregnant ... naturally!

Whether digesting food, making babies or writing a play, how we feel on the inside profoundly affects our results.

When we nourish our emotions, we automatically nourish, balance and strengthen our entire body.

The healing medicine of a mother's love

Dr Lorna Scurfield was one of the greatest inspirations in my life and the lives of many others. A most remarkable doctor and healer, she was the ultimate confidante, friend and above all, wise teacher. What really made her special was her ability to uncover the root causes of physical problems. The following story of hers is a beautiful example of the power of our emotions and tells us so much about the true determinants of health and healing.

One day a young lady in her mid-twenties went to see Lorna. Jenny (not her real name) had all her life been relatively happy, healthy, slim and vital. However, in the months prior to seeing Lorna, she had started to get almost uncontrollable sweet cravings. She was binge eating chocolate, ice-cream and fried food—things that she normally didn't eat much of. She had lost her usual strong desire to exercise, had put on over fifteen kilograms in weight, and was generally feeling pretty depressed. As you would expect, Jenny's central complaint—and overriding goal— was centered on losing weight and getting her energy and motivation back. She wondered whether there might be some special medications, tonics or herbal remedies to stimulate her liver to function normally or help stop her cravings.

Lorna, however, wasn't much into pills or potions. She didn't recommend anything like 'Cut out these foods' or 'Take these tablets or herbs'. Instead, Lorna asked Jenny about her life in general. What was she doing? Had there been any major changes in her life of late? And her favorite question, 'When was the last time you felt really good?'

It turned out that Jenny had always enjoyed a wonderfully close relationship with her mother, from whom she received great emotional support. However, recently Jenny's friends had begun to give her a hard time about how she should move out of home and live on her own. They said she was too old to be living at home with her mother and that she needed to 'grow up'. After a while, despite misgivings, she relented and moved out of home. She moved quite some distance away from her mother and purposely began speaking to her less and less because she thought she had to be more adult, more independent. It was time to be a 'big girl'!

On hearing the sequence of events, Lorna simply recommended ONE THING. She said, 'Jenny, I want you to do one thing and one thing only. I want you to re-establish the close connection, the close bond you had with your mother. If you want to talk with her, call her. If you want to see her, go and see her. Don't 'try' to be grown up or strong. Start following what your heart wants to do, not what your friends want you to do.'

Although Jenny never moved back home, following her consultation she began to ring her mum whenever she wanted to talk. At least once a week they would be on the phone for an hour, sometimes two. Jenny also made a conscious effort to go home to visit her mum as often as she could. She no longer worried about what her friends thought, she just did what she wanted to do, what she felt was right within herself.

You can probably guess where the story ended. Gradually Jenny's sweet cravings began to subside. Instead of chocolate and junk food, she spontaneously desired healthier food and felt like exercising more. Just as quickly as the weight went on, it started to come off. She began to feel like her old self again and never looked back.

While most cases aren't as clear-cut or as easily remedied as this one, it serves as a powerful reminder of the importance of addressing emotional issues before, or together with, physical ones. How often do we create stress for ourselves by putting more importance on what others will think of us than what we think of ourselves? Psychologists often say that whenever we see someone with an ongoing problem—like obesity, anorexia or bulimia—which on the surface seems to relate to food, it usually has nothing to do with food or eating itself. The real issues are emotional or psychological ones, often related to self-esteem, self-love or body image. As with any self-sabotaging behavior, it is usually difficult to change until the underlying emotional issues are addressed.

Most natural health sciences suggest that the tendency to overeat, undereat, smoke, drink alcohol to excess, or engage in other forms of extreme behavior is often just a 'symptom' of an underlying stress or emotional lack.

Natural wisdom suggests that we will have the greatest success in overcoming health compromising behaviors not by trying to change them on the level of willpower, but by nourishing or addressing the underlying emotions that give rise to those behaviors.

Do it now exercise

1. Do you continue to indulge in things you think you shouldn't?
2. Do you find it hard to get motivated to do things you know would be good for you?
3. Are you struggling to achieve a health-related goal by following conventional wisdom?

If so, rather than beating yourself up, just stop for a day or two, and ask yourself what might be behind it all.

Ask yourself:

Is there an underlying or root cause of the problem that I need to address—such as poor self-esteem, boredom, anger over a past event, or stress from having too much work and not enough play?

Do I have some unresolved tension or friction with a partner, friend, family member or work associate?

Is there some other emotional issue present that I need to deal with first?

Emotional health nourishers

While it makes sense that nourishing our emotional health is important, the obvious question is: how do we do it? Ancient health wisdoms, the example of the world's healthiest, metabolize populations, and a growing amount of modern research suggest that three key activities can help.

1. Bliss and the Art of Simple Pleasures

Certain things catch your eye, but pursue only those that capture your heart.

Old Indian saying

What if we were meant to be joyously happy and perfectly contented? What if our natural state was to experience pleasure, joy and bliss? What if suffering first to enjoy later was not Mother Nature's design for us?

Babies, just a few days or weeks old, have no training as to what is good and desirable in this world. Yet babies spontaneously smile, giggle and laugh at even the most mundane things (and in the case of some parents' behavior, the most inane things). Assuming a relatively stress-free pregnancy and birth, the natural state babies are born in is one of wonder, happiness and joy. When we enter this world, we don't have to try to be happy, we don't have to pretend to be happy. In fact, as newborns, we don't even know that there is a happy and a not happy. We are just happy for no particular reason ... until mum and dad forget the nappy thing. It's like we are hardwired for happiness—and maybe we are.

A recent study headed by Dr Lane Strathearn at the Texas Children's Hospital showed that the brain area and circuits which get stimulated when a mother sees her baby smile at her are the same as someone having a drug high.[9] Talk about a natural high. Ask any mother or father to describe 'that feeling' when their own flesh and blood smiles at them unconditionally and they'll suggest there is no greater emotional high. They'll say, 'My heart just melts'. Would they swap it for the most euphoric, ecstasy-producing drug high? Not on your life.

Importantly, it is not just a baby's smile at its mother that elicits what brain researchers call our *'reward pathways'* or our *'pleasure response'.* Any similar experience that warms our heart, makes us smile, gives us an inner glow, sends tingles up our spine, or generally makes us feel good inside produces the same inner 'feel good' chemistry. In fact, there is an almost infinite number of everyday events that can trigger our pleasure response: a lover's embrace, biting into a sweet, juicy fruit, experiencing the sun's first rays, smelling a new season's fragrance. It is as if Mother Nature actually designed us to experience bliss regularly. If we look at these experiences physiologically, such an idea is only strengthened. Neuroscientists tell us that the most advanced part of our brains, the frontal cortex—which less evolved beings don't possess—is literally teeming with receptors for pleasure.

Of course, if we are hardwired for pleasure and bliss, it seems odd that so many of us struggle to experience it. While it can be easy to oversimplify such things, it would seem that the way we have set our goalposts in the modern world is a key contributor. When we buy into the notion that the physical realm of life is more important than the emotional or spiritual level, we can easily be led away from the simple, health-promoting pleasures of life. In seeking the greatest pleasure and most intense bliss, we can easily be brainwashed into believing that they exist in the material world: the perfect job, the ideal relationship, the larger pay cheque, the bigger house. This is all despite research showing us that beyond delivering us basic comforts, more wealth and possessions do not bring any significant improvements in our wellbeing.[10] Ironically, when we stop for just one moment, we often find—as many of the most contented people before us have done—that the most blissful experiences in life are right under our noses. When asked why she lived such a long life, 100-year-old, South Australian-born Maud Young responded, 'I have had such a happy life, I have not had a lot of big things, but I have enjoyed the small things. If I didn't get pleasure out of the small things, then I wouldn't get pleasure ...'[11]

The simple things are always the best

In recent times, science has begun demonstrating that simply having a good laugh can produce effects similar to morphine in reducing pain. If we engage in a passionate interest where we lose a sense of time, we can stimulate our immune system as much as if we are taking the latest immuno-stimulant drug. While most of us would probably not choose to watch Seinfeld reruns instead of having a jab of morphine before major surgery, it is easy to overlook the profound effects such basic, everyday health-promoters can bring.

Doctor Raj Vastrad is one of Australia's leading holistic health specialists and a pioneer in the area of emotional health and healing. In addition to prescribing conventional medications where necessary, Dr Raj focuses on the ancient wisdom of increasing his patients' natural endorphin response as a way of accelerating their body's natural healing system. In one of many similar cases, Dr Raj cited a patient of his ('PK') who had been suffering severe anxiety, depression and social phobia. Social phobia is an anxiety-based condition where one is fearful in social situations. Having relied on anti-depressants and other medication to control his anxiety, after seven months PK was completely medication-free, while reporting a total cessation of anxiety, depression and social phobia. What was the good doctor's prescription?

1. To exercise more. Research clearly indicates that we would need a lot fewer psychiatrists if people simply walked or exercised more.
2. To laugh more. PK was specifically recommended to attend a laughter therapy session once a week, but funny movies or TV shows can work just as well.

3. To devote some time each week to what Dr Raj calls 'P Therapy'—some passion, purpose or personal pleasure.

What did the prescription cost? Next to nothing. Did PK experience any side effects? Indeed he did. He needed fewer drugs, had more
money in his pocket and enjoyed a lot more fun in his life. While not all
cases are as simply remedied as PK's, his story is a powerful reminder
of the profound results we can achieve by reconnecting to the simple,
natural laws of health.

Despite some marvelous advances in modern medicine over the past
few decades, a downside of our drug-dominated medical system is that
we have moved away from many simple, everyday healing practices. In
previous decades, and particularly in traditional medical systems, doctors, medicine men and tribal women healers all knew that the best medicine they carried was not a pharmaceutical pill, the ground root of a plant
or some special herbal elixir. They knew that it was their own *bedside
manner*. A calm, gentle, uplifting and reassuring manner was seen as the
first and foremost healing prescription. An attentive ear and encouraging
words that soothed a patient's heart were known to be as powerful as any
pill or potion. In Ayurveda and most Eastern health sciences, the doctor
is considered as important as the medicine in terms of a patient's healing
prospects. This is because the doctor can uplift the patient's emotions and
inspire hope—or sap their confidence and instill fear.

Modern science itself has shown that the 'placebo effect'—what the
patient feels or believes will happen—is often more powerful than the
medicine itself. Unfortunately, many doctors nowadays are forced to
run their practices as much by the clock as by the heart. Most hospitals
are so focused on fulfilling patient quotas and meeting funding crite-
ria that they can no longer provide what traditionally was considered
the most important patient care. Our beautiful nurses, whose loving
hearts naturally attract them to care for the sick, are commonly so run
off their feet with administrative duties that they scarcely have time for

the consoling words or tender touches that comprise their natural healing instincts and which so many patients yearn for. Ironically, the simple act of touch, which is strongly linked to the emotional heart, has been shown to stimulate our immune system, balance our hormones and activate growth factors. It has been found to be one of the most powerful medicines for returning premature babies to a normal healthy weight, as well as for reducing pain.[12] As many people intuitively know, *a hug a day helps keep the doctor away*.

In 1997, I worked for an aid organization in Cambodia. One of my most precious experiences from that time was how much more physically intimate people there were. Friends, siblings, parents and children would commonly hold each other's hands or walk around arm in arm— including the guys. I even found myself having my hand held or an arm slung around my shoulder by male students at the university I was working at. As an ex-footballer from a traditional 'Aussie bloke' pedigree, I can assure you that the first few times it happened, my heart rate certainly jumped a few notches. However, as I began to learn that this was just a part of the culture, I began to appreciate how beautiful, nourishing and healthy this connection of touch was. Oddly enough, on my return to Australia, my footballing buddies weren't so enamored with my suggestion that we could bond more by holding each other's hands!

> Mother Nature has provided an opportunity for us to receive an abundance of heart medicines within the everyday moments of our lives.
>
> Loving hugs, the words 'I love you', a simple compliment, a child's unbridled laughter, a friend's warm embrace, a mother's consoling touch, engaging in a personal passion—these are all health-promoters par excellence.
>
> All we need to do is stop long enough to enjoy them.

2. Emotional Connection—The Spark of Inner Happiness

A life without friends is like a garden without flowers.

Can you remember seeing a dear friend that you hadn't seen for a long time? Can you remember the feeling that enveloped you in the instant each of you registered the other's presence? In that split second of time, can you remember the inner *spark*, the feeling of connection? Both ancient and modern science tell us that those sparks of connection, whether it be with a friend, a lover or a child, literally shower our bodies with the world's most powerful healing chemistry.

Consider the following.

1. Over one hundred years ago, Wilhelm Roux separated the cells of a frog's eggs in water. Immediately, the cells began to move back towards each other until they eventually reconnected.

2. The first thing individual amoebae (the most basic of life forms) do when separated from their companions is to make their way back to the group.[13]

3. Groundbreaking research done in the United Kingdom during the 1970's found that the presence of an intimate relationship with a husband or partner was the most effective protective factor against psychiatric illness for women. A key factor was that the women felt they could 'share their feelings'. This was independent of whether or not sexual intimacy occurred.[14]

4. A 2002 study of 28,369 male health professionals, reported in the *American Journal of Epidemiology*, showed that men who had higher levels of social integration (e.g. were married, had a large number of friends or relatives, or had strong community involvement) were nearly 20% less likely to die from any cause

than their more 'socially isolated' peers, and almost half as likely to die from coronary heart disease.[15]

5. In 2008, an extraordinary finding from the 20-year Framingham Heart Study social network demonstrated that the relationship between people's happiness extends up to three degrees of separation—that is, to the friends of one's friends' friends. The study found that if someone becomes happy and they have a friend who lives within a mile (about 1.6 km), the probability that the friend is happy increases by 25%.[16] The findings strongly suggest that happiness in part results from the spread of happiness and not just a tendency for people to associate with similar individuals. The study's conclusion was that people's happiness depends on the happiness of others with whom they are connected.

What does all this suggest? It suggests that we are all connected, and that connection is not just good for our health but is critical to it. The desire to connect and be part of a larger whole is built into our emotional and psychological make-up. While we may see ourselves as 'individuals', like the trillions of cells in a body, we are each one cell in a communal body. Without connection, there can be no life. Unfortunately, connecting in our modern world has become an increasingly challenging task. With the ever-increasing pace of life, more of us are catching up on mobile phones, email and internet chat rooms than we are face to face. Online communities are taking over from real communities. The added cost of living means that many mothers have to go back to work almost as soon as their babies are born, while many primary breadwinners feel compelled to work ten, twelve or fourteen-hour days simply to keep up. Spending time with friends, family and loved ones is getting harder and harder. While it is often completely understandable, it can and does affect our health. There is no substitute for real face-to-face, heart-to-heart connections.

In 1965, George Solomon and Rudolph Moos from Stanford University showed an interesting influence on the development of rheumatoid arthritis in women who had a genetic predisposition to the condition. Out of the sample group studied, those who did not get the disease were those considered emotionally healthy. This was on the basis that they were not depressed and 'did not feel isolated or alienated'.[17] Other studies on depression indicate that it is not just associated with negative life events but also lowered subjective social support.[18]

Traditional and indigenous cultures which have survived for tens of thousands of years have lived on the principle that togetherness is the highest virtue. More than even a sense of togetherness, there is a real, concrete, unquestionable appreciation that the community is central to every area of life. A newborn baby is not merely a source of joy and responsibility for the mother or parents, but for the whole tribe or community. Ancient aphorisms such as *'It takes a whole village to raise a baby'* weren't just spoken of but lived by. Conversely, the loss or grief of one was the loss or grief of all.

The traditional Australian Aborigines are a people that I believe represent a tremendous source of ancient wisdom.[a] One of the most integral parts of the Aboriginal native wisdom is their understanding that not only everyone, but also everything, is intimately connected. In 'Voices of the First Day', Robert Lawlor states, 'In the Aboriginal worldview the individual and the collective are the contracted and expanded form of one continuous being'.[19] This worldview expresses itself in the importance they place on both the individual and the collective emotional wellbeing. Lawlor adds, 'Emotions are cultivated in a way that upholds both the spiritual and social order of society'.[20] This further develops into their system of kinship, which goes far beyond our concept of family. One's kin includes not only one's blood relatives but their entire 'skin' relations. A person's father or mother is not just their biological

---

a   While today, we commonly associate Aboriginal communities with various social problems, this is arguably more to do with them being removed from their traditional (natural) way of life. Before they were separated from their traditional foods, sense of purpose and ways of living, they had survived and thrived for tens of thousands of years in relative harmony with each other and their planet.

one, but all their father's brothers and mother's sisters. What this creates is a great web of emotional nourishment. In such communities, the loss of a parent, sibling or child, while still incredibly sad, is not as tragic as it might otherwise be, as within the whole kin, tribe or collective there are many other parents, siblings and children that one can call one's own. Anyone who has had the blessing of being called 'brother' or 'sister' by an Aboriginal elder will know this means much more than some clichéd expression of acquaintance. It is from the heart. It means family.

Today, nearly all wellbeing surveys conducted in various countries around the world show that people who live in country towns or rural communities score far higher on personal wellbeing indexes. Why? Because in these smaller rural and country communities, as in traditional cultures, people connect. Everyone tends to know each other, care for each other and, shock horror, even say hello to each other. God forbid! In 'Healthy at 100', John Robbins talks at length about an American journalist and author named Grace Halsell. Back in the 1970's, she lived for two years with the people of Vilcabamba in the Sacred Valley of the Andes. Vilcabamba has sometimes been called 'the land of eternal youth' and has been the subject of much research as a result of its inhabitants' remarkable health and longevity. While many possibilities have been put forward to explain the Vilcabambans' secret to long life, after living with the *viejos* (the Old Ones), Grace Halsell didn't believe it was the pure waters, the rich soil, the wholesome food, the pristine air or the regular exercise that was the most important factor. She felt that it was their overwhelming '*sense of connectedness*'.[21]

An extension of the importance of connection, and a central factor in nearly all traditional cultures, is the way they respect and treat their elderly. Unlike our youth-obsessed society, where growing old is often associated with becoming less useful and even burdensome, in these cultures the elderly are never ostracized or left to live out their days. The older people get, the more they are glorified, honored, esteemed and looked after. Native American tribes epitomize the wisdom found in all enlightened societies where the elders serve as the moral and spiritual leaders.

Dr Alexander Leaf, in his extensive contact with the long-living peoples of Hunza, Vilcabamba and Abkhasia, noted, 'A striking feature common to all three cultures is the high social status of the aged'. He commented, 'Each of the very elderly persons I saw lived with family and close relatives—often as an extensive household—and occupied a central and privileged position within this group'.[22] Grace Halsell comments on her time in Vilcabamba: 'Living among these people, I learned that it isn't a bank account that can give an old person a sense of security so much as the assurance that he or she never will live alone, nor die alone. Regardless of his age in the Sacred Valley, the Viejo never fears being abandoned or being put away in an institution, unwanted, neglected, left to wither and die'.[23] The Vilcabambans, like the similarly healthy, long-living Abkhasians and Hunzans, place little regard on money and possessions, instead holding their connection to each other as their greatest treasure.

In contrast, within our so-called 'civilized' societies, it is interesting to note the correlation between our eroding sense of community and the rising rates of dementia amongst our elderly citizens. Starting in 2001, researcher Valerie Crooks and her colleagues in Southern California began looking at the possible link between a reduced sense of connectedness and dementia as one ages. 2249 women without dementia began the study and were prospectively interviewed. Their social networks were assessed by the number of friends and family they had, particularly those that they felt they could rely on for help or confide in. Almost twice as many women with small social networks developed dementia as women with larger social networks.[24]

Modern science and traditional wisdom alike suggest that having strong social and support connections should be the most highly prized factors in any health checklist.

Just as high cholesterol, high blood pressure and cigarette smoking are considered risk factors for disease, so should social isolation, communal alienation and loneliness.

Happiness is even more important than a healthy lifestyle

It seems self-evident that connecting with others is good for our health. However, just *how* good is only now being glimpsed by modern science. A nine-year study of over 6900 Californians, ending in the early 1970's, was one of the first to suggest that being happy may be even more important for our health than having a healthy lifestyle.

Headed by Dr Lisa Berkman, the study was aptly titled 'Social networks, host resistance, and mortality'. It looked at the effect that having strong social networks, such as friends, family and partners, had on people's ability to avoid illness and death. Included in the research was whether or not participants followed a conventionally healthy lifestyle by doing things like exercising, eating good food and avoiding smoking. What Dr Berkman found was that people who lacked social and community ties were between two and three times (2.3 for men and 2.8 for women) more likely to die in the follow-up period than those with more extensive contacts. Most intriguing was that the association between social ties and mortality was independent of health practices such as smoking, alcohol consumption, obesity and physical activity.

Those who lived the longest were the individuals who had the highest levels of social connections, regardless of whether they had a healthy or unhealthy lifestyle. Those who followed a healthy lifestyle (e.g. by exercising and managing their weight), but had poor social ties, died sooner.[25]

This study reflects the results of a growing body of scientific research and powerfully demonstrates the main point of this chapter. Although factors like exercising, eating good food and not smoking are vitally important for our health, our emotional health and the experience of love and connection are even more important. Does this mean that we can eat junk food, drink alcohol and smoke whenever we like as long as we have good relationships and social networks? No, that is NOT the case at all. Importantly, Berkman's study also clearly demonstrated that those who lived the longest were the individuals who had both strong social ties and enjoyed a healthy lifestyle. The point is that the inner chemistry of love and connection is a powerful antidote to the stresses of life and can to some degree make up for a less than perfect lifestyle.

> NOTE: Despite the plethora of research showing that those who are married or have good family support or social ties tend to enjoy the best health, it is not marriage or extensive connections per se that are likely to be the key. What matters is whether we are happy. Having a few 'good' friends is more important than having lots of acquaintances, and being 'happily' married is more important than simply being married. (Many of my friends tell me how happily married they are—I just wish I could say the same for their wives!)

The healing power of Fido

For those who may not enjoy strong social connections, there is some good news. It's not just connecting with other people that can help keep us healthy. Mounting research now shows us that connecting with animals, pets or Mother Nature herself can lower our blood pressure, improve our mental health, and help us manufacture the biochemical antidotes to anxiety, stress and depression.

One particular study headed by Dr Rebecca Johnson, Director of the Research Center for Human-Animal Interaction in Columbia, Missouri, showed how just a few minutes of stroking one's dog can build levels of stress-and depression-fighting hormones. In the study, 50 dog owners and 50 non-dog owners spent between 15 and 39 minutes calmly stroking or petting their own dog, a friendly but strange dog, and a robotic dog. Blood pressure was monitored every five minutes and changes in hormones such as serotonin (commonly low in depressed individuals) were assessed. The dogs were tested too!

What were the findings? The blood pressure of the people doing the petting dropped by approximately 10 per cent within 15 to 30 minutes—and their serotonin levels became elevated. Also, in an interesting finding which beautifully highlights the importance of the heart value in our connections, the improvements were found to occur only while individuals were petting their own dog. Serotonin levels failed to increase when owners were petting the strange dog and actually decreased when they were with the robotic dog.[26] Most importantly of all, the dogs' blood pressure dropped immediately upon being petted. (Fido likes his pats.)

Studies in nursing homes with elderly (often lonely) residents, demonstrate profound improvements in their mental health when communal pets are introduced. Other studies have shown that just by looking at puppies, cute babies, dolphins playing or even a beautiful sunset (connecting with nature), we can normalize blood pressure, balance heart rhythms and raise our levels of DHEA. DHEA counterbalances the stress hormone cortisol and is thought to play a key role in resisting disease.

> The most fundamental way we have been designed to nourish our emotional selves is through the experience of positive connection.
>
> If you are low on energy, instead of assuming you need to eat better, consume energy drinks or get more sleep, consider asking yourself whether you just need an emotional recharge by catching up with a friend, playing with a pet, or spending more time with a loved one.

3. CONTRIBUTION—THE MEDICINE OF ALL MEDICINES

If you want happiness for an hour ... take a nap.
If you want happiness for a day ... go fishing.
If you want happiness for a month ... get married.
If you want happiness for a year ... inherit a fortune.
If you want happiness for a lifetime ... help someone else.

Ancient Chinese proverb

While enjoying the simple, everyday joys of life and connecting with others can provide a wonderful source of emotional nourishment, the greatest religious teachers, philosophers and spiritual sages have pointed to an even deeper source of emotional wellbeing. It is based on the law of laws, the one universal natural law which underlies all others:

'As we sow, so shall we reap.'

In the Eastern traditions, '*As we sow, so shall we reap*' is often referred to as '*karma*'. Karma in its essential nature is simply the law of action-reaction. Whatever we put out into the world—positive or negative—comes back to us in equal measure. When a pebble is dropped into a pond, ripples of water spread to the far reaches of the pond and begin to come back. Similarly, the natural health sciences suggest that every thought, feeling and action we give birth to has its own corresponding energy or '*vibration*'. These energetic vibrations, as it were, emanate into our surrounding environment and return to us 'the fruits of our labors'. If our thoughts and actions are positive and life-supporting, the corresponding ripples that return to us will be positive and life-supporting. Thus, according to the eternal law of karma or action-reaction, the greatest thing we can do for our own emotional wellbeing and success is to in some way contribute to the emotional wellbeing or success of others.

Most of us have felt that nice, warm, fuzzy feeling we get when we help someone else. What we don't always appreciate is that this experience may be the greatest medicine we can imbibe. The same areas of our brains that are stimulated during a drug high have also been shown to be activated when we do good deeds. If we could see the internal biochemistry that our bodies manufacture within a split second of doing good, we would witness the natural equivalent of the world's most potent drugs for pain relief, anti-depression and recreational highs. Such an internal cascade of happy chemistry is the basis of the scientific phenomenon known as the *'helper's high.'* This is now a well-known term since researcher Alan Luks surveyed thousands of volunteers and found that those who helped others consistently reported significantly better health than their peers. Sociology Professor Peggy Thoits from Vanderbilt University summarized the findings of a study on volunteer work as follows: '... volunteer work was good for both mental and physical health. People of all ages who volunteered were happier and experienced better physical health and less depression.'[27] Other research has shown positive links between volunteering and improvement in psychological wellbeing, as well as reduction in depression and chronic pain.[28]

Of course, it's not only through volunteering that we can gain the health benefits from helping others—what we could call 'the karma of contribution'. Through a whole host of findings over the last few decades, modern science is now proving to us what we innately know. In whatever form, 'doing good is good for us'. This even applies in the most drastic of cases.

Gay Hendricks is a world-renowned American writer and author in the field of emotional wellness. He recounts a story of a phone call to one of his clients in a neighboring state. The man was really depressed to the point of being suicidal. In looking for ways to help his client move out of his unfortunate state, Gay said to him, 'Is there anything you've seen today that you could do to help someone in need?' His client was silent for a long time before saying that he had noticed that an elderly woman who lives in his apartment building had a whole pile of rubbish that had been slowly accumulating in front of her door. Gay said, 'You don't need to knock on the door or even tell her, but take a broom from your place and go down there and sweep up the mess. I will stay on the phone while you do it'. He said the guy must have been gone for 10 or 15 minutes. Once he started, he couldn't stop and ended up sweeping and cleaning the entire mess. When he returned however, the change in his demeanor was profound. It was like he was '*a completely different person*'.[29]

Medicines of the heart

If your life does not give joy to others, then how can you expect your heart to give any joy to you?

Sri Chinmoy

In traditional cultures as diverse as the American Indians, the Abkhasians of Southern Russia, ancient Vedic civilizations of India through to the Australian Aborigines and countless others, the primary way of contributing to the collective good was through nourishing the hearts of others. These cultures had comprehensive unwritten, and in some cases written, behavioral codes that served as the foundation of all individual and collective life. These 'laws of behavior' were designed to cultivate maximum harmony and good feelings for both the giver and receiver of communication. Importantly, they didn't just cover physical behaviors, but even extended to one's thoughts and feelings.

According to the principle of action-reaction, if we continue to collectively put tonnes of physical pollutants out into our environment, we must expect to eventually pollute ourselves. Similarly, the ancients tell us that if we regularly put out negative or poisonous thoughts (vibrations) about others, we don't just poison them, we also poison ourselves. If you have ever said or done something unpleasant to someone, you may remember experiencing a heavy, churning feeling in the pit of your stomach moments after. In a Native American Indian Code of Ethics it clearly states, 'Avoid hurting other hearts as you would avoid a deadly poison'. Ayurveda outlines a set of *'behavioral rasayanas'*. Rasayanas are things that promote health. Behavioral rasayanas, such as speaking well of others, seeing the good in others and respecting the elderly, are known to nourish our mind, body, heart and emotions.

In his enlightening book, *'The Miracle of Water',* Masura Emoto shows how water crystals change shape when exposed to different words or phrases. When exposed to words such as 'love and gratitude', 'you are beautiful' or 'you can do it', the water molecules take on the most beautiful, pleasing and uniform shapes. But when words such as 'hate', 'you are ugly' or 'you can't do it' are used, the crystal shapes become deformed, unpleasant and unsightly.[30] Interestingly, in relation to the importance of feeling connected to others, Emoto showed that crystals that were ignored suffered more damage than crystals exposed to degrading words. How can all this be, I hear you say? Well, words are extensions of our thoughts, and both our thoughts and the spoken word produce vibrations of energy. Everything is energy, even our subtlest whims and most fleeting feelings. Emoto asserts (and his pictures confirm it) that these vibrations can literally change the vibrational or molecular resonance of water. If this is all true, considering the fact that we are composed of over 70% water ourselves, thinking nice thoughts about ourselves, speaking well of others and focusing on positive, uplifting forms of communication are some of the most critical things we can do for both our own and also others' internal wellbeing. It's not just important to make sure we drink enough water each day, we do well to surround ourselves with emotionally uplifting thoughts and words so that the actual crystal structure of who we are (the water inside us) is most harmonious and health-promoting.

Heart medicines

The following are some simple heart medicine behaviors as encouraged by wise ancient cultures.

1. Greet all strangers and outsiders with a loving heart.
2. Speak the truth … but say it nicely. Ayurveda encourages 'Satyam bruyat priyam bruyat"—'Speak the sweet truth.'
3. Always focus on the good in others. Talk positively about others … even when they're not there!
4. Speak in ways that nourish the emotions. Always seek to uplift and encourage.
5. Treat the young with unconditional love and affection. Respect, honor and learn from the elderly.
6. Focus more on what you can GIVE than what you can receive.
7. As the feeling level of life is most fundamental, keep in mind the simple yet profound words of J. Masai, 'Feelings are everywhere, be gentle.'

Kids, kindness and an antidote to bullying

One of the nicest stories I've ever heard about the simple value of kindness to others was told to me after a seminar I did with a group of Fire Service workers in 2009. After the talk, in which I discussed the importance of nourishing the emotions, a gentleman by the name of Langdon Gould came up to me and said that his son goes to a little primary school just outside Cooma in New South Wales, Australia, called Numeralla Public School. The school has a program where every student is encouraged to do something nice for another student every day without telling them. Each day they are to select a different student.

I was so blown away by this that I contacted the Principal of the school, Ms Jan Rogers, and asked her to explain the program. She said, 'About three years ago, we adopted the Fish Philosophy, which has four simple rules: be there for others, make someone's day, choose your attitude, and play—that is, make learning and interactions with each other fun. One of the parents commented to me that the children in our school are so busy trying to make each other's day that they don't have time to be mean to each other! Students now enjoy a happy, safe and productive learning environment, teachers are able to teach and build positive relationships with their students, and we have a common language that builds community and is inclusive of all.'

So successful has this one little idea been that behavioral problems, bullying and violence, which are becoming widespread at many schools these days, are almost non-existent at this school. Langdon said that sometimes children who have come from other schools attempt bullying tactics. However, if they start trying to bully other kids, they are soon told by the older students that 'we don't do that here'. At Numeralla Public School, the students actually look forward to going to school and doing their good deed each day. Why? Because it makes them feel good![31]

Everyday suggestions for nourishing the emotions

In a modern world of distanced families, diluted communities and hectic lives, nourishing our emotional health can be challenging. However, the wisdom of teachers past and examples of happy, contented individuals suggest there is still much we can do in our day-to-day lives to nourish and strengthen our emotional wellbeing.

Choose joy

While external circumstances can affect our lives and difficulties, sorrows and times of emotional pain will always arise, we generally have an amazing ability to choose our reality. We can focus on things which nourish our emotional health or those that sap our spirit. We can choose to do work that fulfills our heart or work that merely 'pays the bills'. We can choose to focus on what's good in the world or despair at all the injustice. We can choose our attitude each day.

Love thyself

It has been repeated throughout the ages, 'The only true love is self-love'. This of course is not in the egotistical sense, but in the sense that the love of others is really only a reflection of the love we have inside. While connection to others is indeed a powerful medicine, the ancients have declared that loving ourselves is the only love we have complete control over and is what ultimately underpins our emotional state of mind. Loving ourselves regardless of being the right dress size, having the perfect partner or being successful, is the only foolproof way to avoid indulging in behaviors that jeopardize our health. Loving ourselves is the emotional equivalent of eating good quality food.

Transcend

According to ancient Vedic Science, the most profound way to nourish our emotional health is to nourish the level of life that underlies our emotions. This is the non-physical level of life, the level of spirit or consciousness. Enlivening the inner field of consciousness in order to integrate brain activity and culture more balanced and stable emotional functioning is achieved through age-old mental technologies of transcendence. (Transcending is discussed in more detail in Wisdom Six.)

Cultivate a 'no worries' mentality

When social researchers analyze the lives of healthy, long-living people, one of the most consistent findings is that they rarely worry too much about things. We often see this in relationships. Maybe because opposites attract, one partner seems to do all the worrying and the other one doesn't have a care in the world. An elderly couple are interviewed, for example, and the interviewer asks the stress-free partner about their secret to not worrying. The person looks at their partner and, chuckling to themselves, they say, 'She does all the worrying for me' or 'He worries enough for both of us'.

Jeanne Calment, the French woman known throughout the world as the longest recorded living Westerner (she died at 122), said 'If you can't do anything about it, don't worry about it'. So simple, so beautiful, yet so fundamentally wise and true. Much of life we can't change. Much of what we spend so much time and energy worrying about never happens—or is not as bad as we thought. Most importantly, worrying about it never fixes it but merely depletes our joy.

Associate with positive, uplifting people

Do you have certain people, even friends or family, who always want to bring you down or see the worst in any situation? Do others in your life tend to make you feel better about yourself and have a positive, uplifting view of life?

Thoughts have energy and so those you associate with can affect your emotional energy environment. By being around positive people that make you feel good about yourself, you will nourish your emotional environment. Where practical, choose to be with people you enjoy being around and who uplift you emotionally. (While this seems obvious, it's amazing how often we don't do it.) Refuse to associate with people who are constantly negative or critical. If you can't physically ignore or disassociate yourself, do so mentally. Don't be mean or negative yourself, just refuse to buy into their worldview or let their energy drag you down.

Be optimistic but not overly so—follow the Sardinian way

While research generally shows that having an optimistic outlook is good for our health[32], this does not imply that we should necessarily 'try' to have a positive view of life. Forcing or straining goes against the natural tendency of life and thus creates stress. Do you know people who have been to too many self-development seminars and, despite having just become bankrupt, divorced and diagnosed with a life-threatening illness, they still smile and say, 'Isn't life just wonderful'? Ironically, while optimism seems to promote health, rather than being excessively or unnaturally optimistic, many of the world's metabolize people have had a tendency to have an emotional evenness to the highs and lows of life.

In the remote mountainous areas of the Núoro province on the Italian island of Sardinia, there exist a large number of individuals who have lived to over 100 years of age.[33] Three times the Western average in fact. Far from being old and rickety, researchers in the late 1990's found them to be more youthful than many younger Westerners. They still hunted, climbed mountains, cooked and worked with much energy and enthusiasm. Sardinians generally interact in a very uplifting way. This is illustrated by their love of family, laughter and their daily greeting of *'Akentannos,'* which means 'May you live to 100 years'. However, one of the surprising aspects of their way of life is that they are not overly optimistic. With a chequered history of invasion and the like, the Sardinians have become more pragmatic in their ways, responding to good or bad with a similar acceptance.[34]

From a spiritual perspective, equanimity is often more highly valued than positivity. While being optimistic and focusing on the more positive aspects of our lives is undoubtedly a good thing, it should not be strained. We need to be natural. We may do best by focusing on good things and acting with optimistic expectation, but keeping in mind the old adage to *'take it as it comes'*. This sums up the attitude of many contented, long-living people and seems a healthy way to ride the inevitable ups and downs of life.

Make peace with the aging process

Trillions of dollars are made each year on cosmetics, cosmetic surgery and anti-aging pills and potions. All these are based on the belief and expectation that growing older equals more pain and senility and less beauty and value. The process of getting older is a source of so much stress and angst in our society, yet is something that is as natural and inevitable as the setting sun. As the well-aged elders of traditional societies have exhibited, we age best not by fighting the aging process but by making peace with it. We cannot be eternally young in the outer, physical sense and it is not natural to try and do so. Many botched Hollywood facelifts will attest to this!

This is not to say we shouldn't try to stay youthful or to look our best. If modern technology can 'safely' enhance our appearance, that's great. However, if our self-worth is largely governed by things that are destined to deteriorate, we are doomed to a life of emotional anguish and despair. The point is not so much whether we remove our wisdom lines (wrinkles), color our hair (for those who still have some) or even botox our faces (though I'm still to work out how having a forehead that doesn't move when one frowns is a good thing). The critical issue is what type of internal chemistry we create for ourselves by constantly being obsessed with externals.

The toxic effects of a lifetime of worry and anxiety are far more hazardous to our health than any of the toxic chemicals we use in the quest for eternal youth.

Appreciate the spiritual reality that change is the only constant on the material level of life. Day becomes night, summer becomes winter, youth becomes middle-aged, middle-aged becomes older-aged. What is new will be old. What is old will be new.

> Where possible, cultivate the ancient, enlightened way of looking at life as nothing but a never-ending series of cycles, each with its own beauties and lessons.
>
> Refuse to buy into the collective expectation that growing old need be associated with decay or pity. Take inspiration from the long-living people throughout history who have remained purposeful throughout their days and understood that real beauty is found not in how we look but in who we are.

See the funny side of life and don't take things too seriously

The previously mentioned metabolize Westerner, Jeanne Calment, was renowned for her unquenchable sense of humor. Her most famous quip, made on turning 110 was 'I've only ever had one wrinkle and I'm sitting on it'. Dr Alexander Leaf, who studied the world's metabolize cultural groups back in the 1970's, recounted how he interviewed a group of Vilcabambans as part of his search for the secrets to their amazing longevity. The daughter of the oldest Vilcabamban, Miguel Carpio, who was reported to be 123 at the time, was telling Leaf how Miguel still liked to flirt with the ladies and was 'quite a ladies' man in his younger days'. Miguel, knowing everyone was listening, added with a laugh, 'I can't see them too well anymore, but by feeling, I can tell if they are women or not'.[35]

Sometimes in our hectic lives we can forget how important simple pleasures such as having a good laugh can be. However, science confirms that laughter is one of Mother Nature's most profound medicines and it is a common factor in the lives of many healthy, long-living people.

Make time for your passions

At the deepest level, passion and positive emotion are one and the same. Following our passions not only feels good, it is good for us. Mother Nature wants us to be happy and experience joy, and the way she designed us to do this is through our passions.

Make someone's day

In the words of Mark Twain, 'The best way to cheer ourselves up is to try to cheer somebody else up'. If you are feeling a bit flat or stuck in life, consider taking advantage of the karma of contribution by helping someone else in some way. If you don't already, could you do some kind of volunteer work for an hour a month, an hour a week or an hour a day?

The golden rule—nourish yourself first

While it is great to help others, natural wisdom and commonsense (which are basically the same thing) tell us that unless we are feeling good within ourselves, and our own emotional piggy bank is full, we will not feel naturally inclined to support, uplift or help others. It is a basic law of life that unless we love and nourish ourselves first, we can't truly love and nourish others. Nature's wisdom is not to be martyrs. Nourish your emotional needs first and foremost. This is the ground upon which you can provide the greatest service to others and the world.

Question summary—Ideas to help

The following questions can be helpful for staying focused on the everyday activities that most nourish our emotions. If you feel your emotional wellbeing could do with a little boost, look to implement an activity (or activities) in answer to the question that is most pertinent to you.

What is one thing you can do to bring more happiness and joy into your life?

If you lack self-confidence or are regularly self-critical, what is one way that you can love and nourish yourself more?

How can you cultivate more of a 'no worries' mentality or an attitude of 'take it as it comes'?

How can you add more laughter into your days?

How can you spend more time engaging in a personal passion or doing something you love?

What is one thing you can do today to uplift or inspire someone close to you? What can you do tomorrow to make someone's day?

What is the greatest contribution you can make to your family, community or world?

More suggestions on nourishing the emotions have been included in the supplementary ebook—see markbunn.com.au/awmh1_ebook

Seed wisdom

When the heart is at ease, the body is healthy.

Ancient Chinese proverb

We can't truly heal the body without first tending to the heart. Although something might be health-promoting in itself, if doing it creates more stress than joy, it is not truly healthy. If you stress yourself out more in the traffic getting to the gym than you reduce stress by doing your actual workout, don't do it. If following a certain diet or exercise program is so difficult that there is no joy in it for you, don't do it. If you rigidly follow health rules at the expense of doing what makes you happy, don't! When eating, put taste and satisfaction before fats and calories. When exercising, put fun and enjoyment before heart rates and repetitions. In your work or vocation, put purpose and meaning before fancy titles and impressive sounding resumes. In relationships, put pleasure and love before everything else.

We can survive for a long time on a less than ideal diet or less than perfect exercise, however we can't survive for long without happiness in our cells and love in our hearts.

Be healthy, but more importantly, be happy.

Wisdom Two

Live in Tune with Nature's Daily Cycles

For everything there is a season,
and a time for every matter under heaven.
Ecclesiastes 3:1

There is a universal saying in life: 'Timing is everything'.

When trying to conceive a child, timing is everything. When launching a new business product, timing is everything. When telling your wife how the antique vase containing her great-great-grandmother's ashes *accidentally* fell off the mantelpiece during Friday's boys' night, timing is everything!

Similarly, in terms of living a long, healthy life, timing is everything.

Dr Franz Halberg showed that radiation given to mice at certain times of the day can have little physiological effect. However, the same radiation given at the corresponding time at night can kill them. (His results are now used to improve the success of treatments such as chemotherapy.)[1] A local anaesthetic can last about 10 minutes at 8 o'clock in the morning but may last 30 minutes in the middle of the afternoon. No world records in weight-lifting have ever been recorded before noon. Natural births occur at a significantly higher rate between 2am and 6am than at any other time. Heart attacks are three times as common in the morning as they are at night. The reverse is true for asthma attacks. The composition of a mother's breast milk is now known to differ depending on the time of day it is expressed. Breast milk expressed in the morning contains nucleotides that provide a stimulating effect, a bit like caffeine. Breast milk expressed in the evening contains nucleotides that produce a calming, sleep-inducing effect, much like a sedative.[2] Beautiful, isn't it?

The reality is that everything from our DNA to our brainwaves has its own biological rhythm. However, despite many insightful discoveries related to our circadian, or daily rhythms, in terms of our health we still tend to be predominantly consumed with the 'what' or 'how much' of health. We focus almost entirely on how many calories or how much exercise is optimal. In doing so, we overlook the timeless wisdom that 'when' we do things is often even more important.

Common to all traditional cultures has been an appreciation that we humans are intimately connected to the cycles of the sun, moon and universe as a whole, and that living in tune with these cycles is fundamental to our health. Many Native American Indian tribes are known to base their daily and yearly routines around the sun's travels. The traditional Chinese understanding of opposites—*yin and yang*—which underpins all that they do, can be seen in the opposing yet harmonious relationship of the sun and moon, night and day. The third principle of ancient Mayan medicine was the recognition of natural cycles. Such cultures knew that there are specific times to plant and specific times to harvest, specific times to eat heavy foods and specific times to eat light foods, specific times to be active and specific times to rest. Even in today's well-researched longevity hotspots such as Hunza, Abkhasia, Vilcabamba and Campodimele, the relative absence of modern-day technology and industrialization has meant that they have naturally lived in close alignment to the eternal cycles of night and day.

> Fundamental to the natural world is a number of immutable cycles and rhythms.
>
> As we are intimately connected to the natural world ourselves, we either support or compromise our health by living in tune with or going against these eternal rhythms.

Nature's daily clock

In looking to understand the cycles of nature that promote the highest levels of health—and that have been followed by the world's healthiest, metabolize peoples—we need to look beyond the modern scientific analysis of biochemicals, hormones or body temperatures. We need to look to the deeper wisdoms of life. We need to look to the holistic intelligence that governs our entire universe. Fortunately, ancient sciences have preserved such knowledge in exquisite detail. The Ayurvedic sages detailed exactly how Mother Nature's unseen intelligence expresses itself in the cycles and rhythms of life through what's known as the 'doshas'. The doshas are understood to be the basic, underlying principles of intelligence that govern all of life. From the wind to the mountains, from the earth to the outer solar systems, from our individual human lives to the various cycles that underlie our natural world, the doshas are at work. Each dosha, of which there are three in number, has unique qualities and governs different times of the day, month and year according to these qualities. The dosha known as 'Vata' is light, spacey and airy, like the *wind*. 'Pitta' is hot, dynamic and intense, like *fire*. 'Kapha' is slow, heavy and more *earthy*. According to Ayurveda, our 24-hour daily clock is made up of six interconnected four-hour cycles. Each of these cycles is governed by a particular dosha (underlying principle) which supports specific physiological functions. Either consciously or unconsciously, individuals and cultures that have tended to resist illness and enjoy relatively disease-free lives have understood that certain activities best support the internal functioning of the body according to the different times of the day. We will look at each of these times or cycles in detail.

NOTE:

1. You do not need to understand the doshas in detail. They are simply mentioned in order that you may better appreciate why certain recommendations apply at certain times.
2. The times shown are approximate and can vary slightly with the cycles of sunrise and sunset.
3. While it would seem obvious to start with the morning cycle, many of us do not feel naturally motivated to do what Mother Nature designed us to do in the morning hours. This is because our nightly routines typically violate the natural laws of health. For this reason, we will begin from the evening cycle as this will help you to wake up refreshed, energized and motivated—just as Mother Nature intended.
4. Do not stress yourself if you cannot immediately align your lifestyle with all of the following recommendations. It is an almost inevitable part of Western society that to function in it, we cannot always enjoy the ideal daily routine nature designed for us. Do the best you can, but don't strain. Never forget, enjoying life is number one.

THE EVENING CYCLE (6PM–10PM)—EATING LIGHT AND SLOWING DOWN

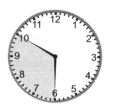

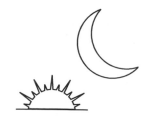

Imagine a beautiful lotus flower fully open during the day. Then, in your mind's eye, see it slowly closing down as the dark of night descends, culminating in being fully closed by the evening. This is symbolic of Mother Nature's universal transition from the dynamic activity of the day to the resting phase of the night. It is also symbolic of the changes that occur within us. As the sun begins to set and day shifts towards night, Mother Nature starts to slow down in readiness for her night cycle. From around 6pm, the earthy (Kapha) qualities of heaviness and slowness begin to take over. This period is designed to wind us down from the incessant activity of the day. As the sun or 'universal fire' goes down, so too our digestive fire, and indeed all our internal organs, organ channels, nervous system and biological systems start to retire for the evening. Like the lotus, everything closes down in order to take full advantage of the peak cleansing and rejuvenation cycle that follows— the 10pm to 2am cycle.

The evening meal—a key to super energy, good sleep and weight loss ... or to sickness and suffering

Food that we do not digest by the time we go to bed sows the seeds of sickness and disease.

If there was a pill that could give us up to 50% more energy, significantly reduce our risk of chronic disease and almost guarantee a healthy weight for the rest of our life, many people would probably pay hundreds if not thousands of dollars for it. Ironically, 90–95% of us (Westerners) do something each and every day that, if changed, could deliver all the above benefits and more. It doesn't take any more time out of one's day, actually saves money, and is a hallmark of the healthiest, metabolize people throughout time. It is the most basic, simple, yet rarely followed wisdom of *'eating light at night'.*

As human beings, we are just not designed to eat much in the evening. We are designed to eat our main meal in the middle of the day.

This is when the sun and our digestive fire are at their peak. Just as the sun sets in the evening and disappears by nightfall, our inner digestive sun, or 'fire', also sets. Think of a dynamic, blazing campfire that slowly dwindles in strength until it is just a bed of hot embers. This is similar to how our digestive fire lessens in strength from daytime to nighttime. After sunset, our digestion, along with all its related internal processes, moves into its resting phase in order to facilitate the next cycle of inner purification during sleep.

The ancients knew that eating lightly at night was the secret to 'the sleep of the gods'. When we do this, our body can fully focus its energies on eliminating the impurities and stresses that have accumulated during the day. Without the burden of a big evening meal to digest, we are better able to repair, revitalize and rejuvenate ourselves and so wake up as Mother Nature intended: with the birds—bright, energized and motivated.

But what do we do? Most of us come home at 7, 8 or 9 o'clock at night and sit down to our main meal of the day. Steak and three veg. Chicken parmagiana that's falling over the sides of the plate. Spaghetti bolognese with a side of chips. And would we like some ice-cream, a little slice of cheesecake or some apple pie just to top it off? Well, it would be rude not to. There are children starving in other countries, so it wouldn't be right not to eat everything that's in front of us! So we loosen our belts, dig in and eat until we feel like we're about to give birth. When we do this, instead of waking up 'bouncing out of bed with the birds', we wake up heavy, dull and sluggish. We need two alarm clocks, a hot shower and three cups of coffee just to get ourselves into the land of the living. Of course, rather than believe that we might actually have anything to do with it, we simply blame our 'slow metabolism' and rationalize it all by declaring, 'Oh, I'm just not a morning person.'

Though modern science has historically been more concerned with the old calories-in and calories-out understanding of weight management, a recent Northwestern University study has shown the first causal evidence linking meal timing to increased weight gain. The study, headed by Fred Turek, Director of the Center for Sleep and Circadian Biology, found that mice that ate at irregular times—the equivalent of the middle of the night for humans—put on almost two-and-a-half times more weight than mice eating the same type and same amount of food during naturally wakeful hours (48 percent compared to 20 percent).[4] Turek said, 'How or why a person gains weight is very complicated, but it clearly is not just calories in and calories out'. On summing up the study's findings, he poignantly commented, 'Better timing of meals ... could be a critical element in slowing the ever-increasing incidence of obesity'.

All of this has of course been known for thousands of years in the Eastern traditions. Ayurveda tells us that large, heavy meals at night are not only likely to be poorly digested (as our internal fire is not so strong), but totally compromise our nightly rejuvenation cycle. Instead of our body's resources going to help our brains revitalize, our livers detox and our muscles rejuvenate, they are diverted to our stomachs to try and digest the three-inch steak, the cheesy parmagiana or the chocolate pudding. Even worse, improperly digested food, known as 'ama' in Ayurveda, is not always easily removed from our bodies. Unless eliminated, such incompletely digested food accumulates night after night in our cells and tissues. Over time, this undigested mush starts blocking vital internal channels and impairing cellular communication. The ancient Ayurvedic texts clearly detail how ama directly leads to weight gain, joint stiffness, mental lethargy and a host of other imbalances. Indeed, improperly digested food or ama is said to be *'the bed of all disorders'* as it blocks the natural flow of intelligence that underpins its proper functioning.

While modern science does not have this understanding, sticky residues or 'plaques' are known to interfere with many internal processes. Atherosclerotic plaque is what lines our arteries. Plaques build up in our joints and play roles in certain types of arthritis. Parkinson's disease, Alzheimer's disease and other forms of dementia are commonly associated with plaques that build up between the neurons or communication channels of our brains. The normal flow of communication gets blocked and as a result all areas of mental functioning—memory, clear thinking, decision-making—begin to deteriorate. The question is, where do these plaques come from? Modern medicine does not really know. Enlightened medicine men and women of times past knew that the main cause of these plaques is the improper digestion of food. Every part of our bodies is, after all, nothing other than the food we have eaten. One of the most common ways we do this is by eating heavy or late dinners when our digestive fire is generally weak and less able to properly process food. It is well documented that one of the most significant differences between the diets of long-living people from traditional cultures and our own is that they eat far fewer calories per day. The Hunzans, for example, typically consume 500 to 1000 fewer calories per day than the average person in America. More importantly, most of their calories are consumed during the active, daylight hours, when digestion is strongest.

Wise ancient cultures who lived in harmony with the natural cycles knew to eat sparingly, if at all, once the sun went down. This is why traditionally the evening meal was known as 'supper'. If one did eat after sunset it was only something that could be 'sipped' or 'supped'. Why do we need a big meal at night anyway? We're about to go to sleep!

> The ancient sciences tell us that all health conditions—from obesity to heart disease—are substantially aggravated (and in some cases even instigated) by violating the most basic of natural laws—eating our largest, heaviest meal after sunset.

Don's 'eat light at night' transformation

For almost two years back in the late 1990's, I had the opportunity to travel around Australia with a team of Maharishi Ayurvedic doctors. Sitting in on hundreds of health consultations, I saw a wide variety of people from all walks of life. People came with everything from minor aches and pains through to serious medical conditions such as recent heart attacks, diabetes, irritable bowel syndrome, chronic fatigue and various types of cancer.

One of the most common behaviors in the majority of patients was their practice of eating their main meal at night. Getting to see many of the same people every three months brought home the power of simply eating light at night. Once people changed their routine to eating smaller, more easily digested evening meals, their health would typically be transformed. Weight would fall off, energy would skyrocket and 'morningitis' (my term for not being able to get out of bed without an alarm clock before 7am) would vanish. Even conditions such as arthritis and chronic hypertension would commonly decrease or even disappear.

One of the most drastic transformations I can recall was a guy called Don. He was in his mid-50s, a good 20 kg overweight with high blood pressure, high cholesterol and an obvious hot temper. Being semi-retired, many of his days were spent playing golf. Even more of his days were spent at the 19th hole (the clubhouse), socializing and enjoying a few drinks. Don was like many men. He wanted to lose weight but didn't want to know anything about reducing his alcohol intake or his consumption of good food. When asked about his typical daily food intake, Don replied that most days he played golf in the morning and then had a big, 'long' lunch at the club. When he got home at night, he ate whatever his wife had cooked for dinner. When asked if he was hungry at dinnertime, he responded, 'No, not really. But Mary loves to cook, and the evening meal is her main meal and the family meal, so I wouldn't want to offend her by not eating.'

Don's initial prescription was pretty simple. He didn't have to change what he did at lunchtime, but he was instructed that dinner was to be totally determined by his appetite. If he wasn't hungry, he was just to have a very light supper or nothing at all. If he didn't have such a big lunch and was somewhat hungry in the evening, he could eat moderately but was to avoid heavy, hard-to-digest foods such as heavy meats, rich desserts, cheese or nuts. Don was quite happy with this. He was not really hungry in the evening anyway and, as it turned out, Mary was quite relieved even happy—that she no longer had to cook a big meal at night. Anyway, she too was in the process of changing her main meal to lunchtime.

While struggling a little initially, Don got into the habit of just having a small supper at night. Occasionally after a big lunch at the club, he skipped dinner altogether. This one change brought about remarkable results. Each time Don came back for a follow-up consultation, there was one less notch on his belt buckle. He said his energy 'had gone through the roof' and after just three months, his cholesterol and blood pressure were just about back in the healthy range. While he wouldn't admit to noticing any dramatic changes emotionally, his face was a little more relaxed and clear each time he came back. He was much nicer to deal with, his temper had mellowed, and he began to laugh more. Mary actually said that his children and some golfing buddies of his were asking her, 'What's happened to Don?'

One could well ask, 'How can eating lighter at night improve one's emotions or temperament?' In Ayurveda and many of the Eastern health sciences, it is suggested that just as our bodies have to process the food we eat, they have to process our emotional experiences too. By eating lightly at night, we not only allow our internal organs, such as our liver, to process any alcohol and fatty foods consumed during the day, we also promote the effective digestion and elimination of any unhealthy or toxic emotional residues. Without having to also contend with heavy food in our stomach, our bodies are better able to process toxins such as alcohol and purify themselves physically, mentally and emotionally.

As if it were yesterday, I remember the day about nine months after Don first came in. Putting on a well-rehearsed, yet tongue-in-cheek act of being extremely upset, he brought in an old pair of trousers. Waving a small white docket in his hand, he screamed, 'What have you done? You've cost me a fortune. Not one piece of my clothing fits me anymore. I've had to go and buy a whole new wardrobe, so here is the bill.'

This example further brings home the folly of counting calories. Not all calories are the same.

> More important than how many calories we eat is whether we properly digest the calories (food) we eat.
>
> The time of day we eat those calories, i.e. day or night, is far more critical for our health and our waistlines than blindly eating some arbitrary number of calories each day.
>
> If you really want to lose weight, don't follow complicated, confusing calorie counting. Follow the natural laws of health and simply eat less at night.

Eating light at night—Ideas to help

If the evening meal is your family meal, it is certainly great to continue this. The emotional benefits of eating as a family are priceless. However, you can still catch up with the family without having to eat a big, heavy meal that compromises everyone's health. Simply vary your meal choices to favor lighter, more easily digested foods or gradually reduce the size of your meals. Focus more on the conversation than the food.

Don't feel that you necessarily have to change your dinner menu. To begin with, just cut down the serving sizes of heavy, hard-to-digest foods and favor lighter foods (see Table 1). For example, start by cutting down your portion of meat to half or three-quarters and add in more rice or vegetables.

Gradually substitute a heavy meal with a light meal variation one or two nights a week. For example, fish and vegetables instead of steak and chips or a vegetable stir-fry instead of chicken pasta with cheese sauce.

When eating out, consider one of the following—having one or two courses rather than three, having an entrée size serving for main course, skipping the entrée, going halves in dessert with a friend.

If you are trying to lose weight, rather than eating potentially health-compromising 'low carb' diets at night, simply eat less food. (More on low carb diets, as well as further suggestions and meal ideas for eating lighter at night, have been included in the supplementary ebook at markbunn.com.au/awmh1_ebook)

As with all meals, the most important factor to consider at the evening meal is simply to eat according to your appetite. In line with this, keep the following guideline in mind when determining whether your evening meal size is suitable.

If you wake up in the morning feeling light, clear and refreshed, generally speaking your evening meal was appropriate.

If you sleep well but wake up feeling heavy, dull or slow to get going, lighten your evening meal and/or eat earlier.

Table 1: Examples of heavy and light foods

Heavy	Medium	Light
most meats— particularly beef, lamb, pork (chicken, turkey less so) heavy sweets— chocolate, cream cakes, cheesecake hard cheeses nuts	fish soft cheeses (e.g. ricotta) raw vegetables/salads sweet biscuits bananas potato / sweet potato	cooked vegetables soups dry roasted rice dhal (cooked lentils) cous cous, semolina, noodles small servings of heavier foods

* In terms of the evening meal, heavier foods would be avoided or reduced and lighter foods favored.

The early evening switch-off—the key to settled sleep

Another key difference between cultures where a high percentage of citizens live long, sprightly lives and our own can be seen in what we each do after the sun sets. Without late-night shopping, 10pm happy hour or the world wide web, people from traditional cultures have automatically been more connected to the natural waves of rest that descend upon us in the evening hours. Just as the great majority of animals in the forest wind down after sunset, the heavier, slower qualities that increase within us at this time are encouraging us to do the same. If you have ever been camping and can remember sitting around a campfire telling stories at night, you can probably remember the natural wave of heaviness that came upon you as night descended. This is Mother Nature's balm. This is her encouraging tap on the shoulder that it is time for us to begin our 'resting' phase of the cosmic cycle, i.e. to prepare for sleep.

The fact that so many in our society can't sleep, and that sleep problems cost developed countries billions of dollars a year in health-related expenses and lost productivity, tells us that something is seriously wrong with our relationship with the natural cycles.

While we spend millions on pills, potions, herbal supplements, state-of-the-art laboratory testing, specially designed beds, pillows and even sleep machines that cost more than the average car, getting restful, rejuvenative sleep was never meant to be difficult. As far as we know, animals in the forest do not toss and turn in an attempt to get to sleep. Grizzly bears don't wake up in the morning and ask their partners, 'How did you sleep, honey?' Without modern-day technology to distract them from their natural cycles, getting to sleep and staying asleep is a given. It's as natural as breathing.

While our modern 24/7 style of living can make nighttime activity much more exciting, it can have its downside. Instead of slowing down with the start of our natural sleep wave (which begins around 7pm), we are easily tempted to work later, exercise later and socialize later. Even what we do to relax at night can stimulate more than calm us. This may include surfing the web, playing computer games or watching high-action TV. These can provide an all-important mental break from the day's activities, however they can also counteract our body's natural desire to slow down, over-activate our nervous systems and hamper our ability to sleep when we are designed to.

For those who find getting a good night's sleep difficult, ensuring a marked reduction of physical and mental activity from around 7pm is a good place to start. Light, relaxing activities that promote a settled and calm mind are generally best at this time. While many traditional cultures dedicate this time to telling the stories of their land or honoring their gods, for us, pleasant (non-work based) conversations, quiet reading or TV that is light and relaxing rather than highly stimulating can work well. Such activities allow us to tune in to our body's first signals of wanting to go to sleep, which usually come before 10pm.

THE NIGHT CYCLE (10PM–2AM)—THE PEAK WAVE OF INNER CLEANSING AND REJUVENATION

   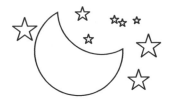

Early to bed, early to rise makes a man healthy, wealthy and wise.

I am the first to admit that the idea of regularly going to bed early is rather boring and unglamorous. In fact, it is so obvious, and we have all heard it said so often, that it seems a complete waste of time to mention it again. I could of course tell you far more interesting things like how cocoa, as domesticated by the ancient Mayans, can be used to help reduce heart disease and stroke. I could go on about how the sap from the native Indian guggul tree is now being used to treat obesity and high cholesterol. Or I could explain how drinking cow's urine is now being put forward as a promising treatment for diabetes (seriously!). These would all be very interesting. However, while being far less newsworthy, every night we have access to the most profound, natural means of reducing heart disease, stroke, obesity, high cholesterol and diabetes ever invented. The fact is, simply sleeping when Mother Nature designed us to does more to detox, de-stress, rejuvenate and revitalize our minds and bodies than any wonder pill or new-age herbal medicine ever will.

The ancients understood that the natural cycle from 10pm–2am is the most critical of all in terms of our lifelong health and wellbeing. Importantly, it is also the cycle that is most abused in our modern society and closely connected to the majority of common health problems people face. In Ayurveda, this cycle is known as the second 'fire' (Pitta) cycle. Have you ever noticed that when you stay up during this period, you can suddenly become ravenously hungry around midnight? This is often known as getting the '*midnight munchies*'. Being right in the middle of this cycle, it is an interesting indicator of increased fire at work. However, this period of increased fire is not designed for digesting potato chips, cream puffs or pizza. Whereas the corresponding period during the day is designed for digesting food to provide us with energy and vitality, the purpose of the corresponding nighttime cycle is to digest any impurities and fatigue that we have accumulated during the day.

> Between 10pm and 2am is the time when our bodies are at their peak capacity for repairing cells, dissolving stress, eliminating toxins (detoxifying), and generally rejuvenating our entire system.
>
> To maximize this internal rejuvenation and cleansing, ideally it is a time when we are 'asleep'!

It's not just the quantity of sleep (how much) but the quality (when we get it)

Have you ever heard the old wives' tale, 'An hour before midnight is worth two after'? Maybe your grandmother used to say it. If she did, perhaps you thought she was smoking something or had forgotten to take her medication. However, that little old wives' tale is actually based on a universal, ancient truth. In terms of the inner rejuvenation and cleansing cycles of our bodies, it is 100% accurate.

While modern science focuses almost entirely on how much sleep we get, that's only half of Mother Nature's recipe for revitalizing sleep. You may have noticed that sleeping eight hours from midnight to 8am will generally leave you waking up heavy, sluggish and slow to get going. However, eight hours' sleep from 10pm to 6am will generally have you feeling light, refreshed and bouncing out of bed. The reason for this is that from 10pm we take full advantage of our bodies' four-hour peak rejuvenation cycle. We ride the wave of inner purification and revitalization while it's at its maximum power. The later we go to bed, the more we miss this wave and the more likely stress, fatigue, impurities and toxins will accumulate in our cells. While few of us want to be in bed before 10pm each night, regularly violating such a fundamental law of nature must *by law* bring about problems. Cultures that have been scientifically studied for having large numbers of centenarians and or significantly reduced incidence of chronic disease typically go to sleep early in the night cycle.[4] University of Rome researchers studying the longevity of people from Campodimele (the hilltop village in southern Italy known as Europe's 'village of eternal youth') noted that in addition to being very closely aligned to the natural daily cycles in general, they regularly went to bed soon after dusk.[5]

If you were asked to guess the key lifestyle causes of obesity, diabetes, heart disease and stroke, you might reasonably suggest diet, exercise and possibly stress. They are all certainly true enough. However, one commonly overlooked lifestyle factor is insufficient or poor quality sleep, which is now being correlated just as strongly with nearly every major Western disease. Lack of sufficient quality sleep is not just a case of feeling a bit tired or not quite performing at our peak, it can literally kill us!

In late 2007, a Working Group of the International Agency for Research on Cancer, a branch of the World Health Organization, concluded that 'shiftwork that involves circadian disruption is probably carcinogenic to humans'.[6] Let me repeat that in layman's terms. Based on human and animal studies to date, shiftwork, where the body's natural rhythms are routinely disrupted, is a probable cancer-causing agent. While this suggestion may seem extreme, it's perfectly plausible when viewed in the light of the natural laws of health. In fact, one need look no further than the vast and unambiguous research on the health and performance of night shiftworkers to see that there really is little argument that we humans are designed to be asleep at night. As compared to the general population, shiftworkers are well known to suffer a far higher incidence of heart problems, weight disturbances, anxiety, nervous system troubles, accidents, sleep apnea and many other health disorders.[7]

They don't call it (nightshift) the 'graveyard' shift for nothing.

While it's good to be sympathetic to those who do shiftwork longterm, the point here is that it's not simply working at night that compromises our health. Regularly staying up late to play computer games, grab some bargains on ebay, or watch 'Saturday Night Live' will similarly disrupt our delicately balanced internal cycles. More and more good science is now showing links between a whole host of serious health problems and poor quality sleep, insufficient sleep or being exposed to light during the nighttime hours. Just some of these include heart disease, breast cancer, autoimmune disorders including rheumatoid arthritis (inflammation), weight gain (obesity), type 2 diabetes, and ADHD and behavioral problems in children.[8] (11 studies listed)

Although some scientists would caution that this research is as yet inconclusive, from the law of commonsense and the ancient wisdoms of health, it's a no-brainer. Sleep, particularly between 10pm and 2am, is where our bodies repair, rejuvenate, eliminate fatigue and process most of the impurities built up during the day. If we skimp on sleep during our body's peak rejuvenation time, we won't process excess fats and impurities as effectively. Thus weight gain must be more likely. If we don't repair our tissues and neutralize unwanted metabolic by-products as effectively, arterial plaques and heart disease must be more likely. If we don't eliminate excess sugars and revitalize our pancreas effectively, our chances of diabetes must increase. When we miss our body's primary wave of repair and revitalization, we also won't rebalance vital hormones, restore optimal energy levels, strengthen our immune systems or support our body's general self-healing mechanisms as effectively. It's not rocket science. It's simple, basic, natural wisdom. While researchers and authors who report on the factors behind the lives of the world's healthiest and metabolize people typically point to their healthy whole food diets, regular exercise and happy home lives, their habit of sleeping in tune with the natural cycles is undoubtedly just as important.

Although boring, unglamorous and often just downright difficult, the undeniable, age-old truth remains that for optimal health, the best time for getting to sleep is early in the night cycle.

To promote robust health and longevity, take advantage of your body's peak rejuvenation cycle.

Eat light dinners and get to bed early—by 10.00 or 10.30pm—most nights.[a]

THE EARLY MORNING CYCLE (2AM–6AM)—ZOMBIE TIME, WASTE DISPOSAL & WAKE-UP

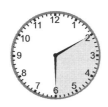 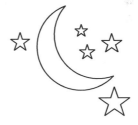

Further evidence that we humans are supposed to be resting rather than working or playing during the nighttime hours is illustrated by what nightshift workers commonly call 'zombie time'. Zombie time runs from around 3am to 6am. The more scientific term is the 'circadian nadir'— 'circadian' referring to the 'daily cycles' and 'nadir' meaning 'low point'. This is the time when most of our physiological cycles, other than those related to repair and revitalization, are at their lowest levels of functioning. Though some studies in certain areas have found no difference in the number of accidents caused by human error related to the time of day or night[9], it is no coincidence that the vast majority show a strong correlation between nighttime activity and an increase in human error accidents. The Chernobyl and Three Mile Island nuclear disasters and the Exxon Valdez oil tanker spill were significant human error disasters, all made in 'zombie time'. Clearly, it is not a time for high-level performance.

---

a   These times obviously do not apply to children, where earlier bed times are more favorable—depending on age.

In the Ayurvedic scheme of things, the natural purpose of the 2am—6am cycle is to complete the internal cleansing and rejuvenation work begun in the previous cycle. Rapid eye movement (REM) activity associated with dreaming is common at this time. This helps reinvigorate and restore optimal brain functioning. When we are well-rested through this phase, all impurities and toxins can be properly processed and our bodies can start the new day with a clean slate. Assuming we are in balance and have followed the previous day's cycles, sometime just before or not long after sunrise is when we are naturally designed to wake up. The exact time depends on our individual constitution, but just as when the animals in the forest start waking up, the birds start chirping and the roosters start crowing, we humans are also designed to start our day close to dawn. In Ayurveda, the early morning cycle is known to be governed by the qualities of space, air and lightness (Vata). Thus, when we arise during this time, assuming we have gone to bed at a reasonable time, we will naturally wake up feeling light, flexible and energized.

'But I'm just not a morning person!'

If you are someone who comes alive at night and regards 'sleeping in' as the most hallowed activity in life, you are unlikely to be too impressed with the assertion that we are designed to arise early. If you are a typical night person, you might reply, 'Yes, that's all good in theory, but I'm a night owl. I just don't function well in the mornings. I am definitely not a morning person.' End of statement!

Unfortunately, according to the eternal laws of nature, there is no such thing as 'night people'. For those who might disagree, doing the following little experiment usually proves the fact. Come home one night and pretend you were living in the early 1900's. Eat a light, early dinner. Turn off your computer, TV, radio, iPod, electric clocks and any other high-stimulation electronic devices. Take off your watch, turn off any extraneous lights and keep your other lights dimmed. If you have kids, put them to bed early and simply read, listen to soft music or engage in relaxing conversation. Most importantly, make a point of going to bed as soon as you feel the urge. Without artificial lighting, TV, radios or computers to overshadow your natural desire for sleep—unless you have a chronic imbalance—you will almost certainly be asleep by 9.00 or 9.30pm the first night. If you repeat the same routine for another one or two nights, you may even be asleep by 8.00 or 8:30pm, along with all other diurnal animals. You will also wake up early, with the birds, and feel fantastic! The effects would be even more dramatic if you did the same process out in nature or in the bush.

As humans, we are all governed by the same cycles and rhythms of nature. Our whole biological and physiological functioning is set within the rhythms of the day and night cycles and the corresponding cycles of light and dark. While it is true that some people do have a constitutional predisposition to being slower in the mornings, this does not make them night people or 'not morning people'. The reason some people think they are not morning people has little to with genetics or bad luck. It is almost always due to some violation of the natural laws of health. The most common of these include:

i) Eating heavy dinners late at night

As discussed, sleeping can only provide its optimal rejuvenative benefits if we have minimal food in our stomach. If we have just dined out at the all-you-can-eat buffet or ravished a triple chocolate fudge sundae not long before we hit the sack, we can forget about waking up feeling like a morning person.

ii) Sleeping out of sync with the natural cycles

Supposed night owls naturally tend to stay up later at night. This of course means they get less sleep during the peak rejuvenation cycle (the 10pm—2am cycle). They are also more likely to sleep well into the morning cycle. Both of these factors promote waking up heavier, less revitalized and the opposite of a morning person.

iii) Sleep deficit

If we have built up a sleep deficit by getting inadequate or poor quality sleep over a period of time, even having one good night's sleep can result in waking up with residual fatigue or tiredness. This obviously does not mean we are 'not a morning person', it just means we need to get more sleep, more regularly, at the right time of night.

Marita West, a Performance and Improvement Coordinator at Logan City Council in Queensland, Australia, attended a talk I gave to her work group in May 2009. Rarely waking up fully energized or bright in the mornings, she summed up what so many people experience when changing their evening routine. Just three days after the talk, she sent me an email that read: 'Mark, I started changing my lifestyle, especially my eating patterns, to align with the natural cycles. My sleep has improved out of sight. I have been bouncing out of bed at 5.30am each morning—pretty sad really (her words)—and haven't felt at all heavy or lethargic since.'

Some people skimp on adequate sleep for years, eat three-course banquet-type dinners until 9 o'clock at night, repeatedly go to bed late and say, 'I don't know why but I'm just no good in the mornings.' Hmmmm.

The fact is, we are all morning people to greater or lesser degrees. The confusion is not one of genetics, it is one of lifestyle and violation of the fundamental laws of life.

THE MORNING CYCLE (6AM–10AM)—ELIMINATION, EXERCISE AND BREAKFAST

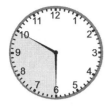

There is no hope for a civilization which starts each day to the sound of an alarm clock.

Source unknown

The morning cycle that starts each new day is governed by the same heavier, slower and earthier qualities that begin each night cycle. While sleeping in is a much-cherished pastime in our culture, especially after a late night or three, we are far more likely to feel heavy and lethargic the entire day by doing this. This is due to the fact that our bodies go into a different cycle after 6am and this applies regardless of how many hours of sleep we get. Instead of arising with the space and air qualities of the preceding Vata cycle, we arise with the heaviness of the earthy Kapha cycle. More than just feeling heavy, we are also far more likely to gain weight or to struggle to lose weight the longer we sleep in after sunrise. Unfortunately, this cycle is one we were never designed to be regularly sleeping through.

If our previous day's routine has been in accord with the daily cycles, we will generally wake around sunrise. Our bodies will have completed the processes of food digestion, tissue repair and cellular refuelling as well as accumulating and transporting any wastes off to our 'waste dis-posal unit'. Like the perfectly orderly mechanics of a clock, right at the junction point between the end of the nighttime cleansing cycle and the new day dawning, our bodies are naturally primed for their first as-signment of the day—*major evacuations!* Generally, if everything is in balance, we will have the urge to eliminate during this time. Be alert to any *pressing* matters, and at your first prompting complete this most important function.

Constipation consternation

How many happy, constipated people do you know? While we tend to have a good laugh about such matters in the West (which is quite funny when it's not me—don't get me wrong), if things do not regularly move down there, it's no laughing matter.

In natural health-care systems, such as Ayurvedic medicine, Traditional Chinese medicine and Tibetan medicine, our bodies are seen as a flow of energy. On an even deeper level, Ayurveda explains it as a 'flow of intelligence'. The natural flow of energy or intelligence in the area of our intestines and bowel is ideally in a downward direction. Any blockage or impaired functioning in this region can significantly disturb this natural flow. Like a tennis ball that hits the ground and thus bounces back up, energy that can't move down due to some obstruction will tend to have its flow reversed, i.e. the energy flow is forced upwards. In the case of obstructions in the bowel region, this upward energy flow can begin interfering with the proper functioning of important organs above it, such as the kidneys, spleen, liver, stomach, pancreas and heart.

> In most time-tested natural health systems as well as from modern medicine's own recent findings, blocked energy flow due to repeated obstruction or ineffective elimination of waste matter from the bowels can contribute to more serious problems such as chest or head pain, general bowel disease, diverticulosis, irritable bowel syndrome and possibly even bowel cancers.

Being *'a bit stuck'*, or regularly failing to eliminate within the morning cycle, is not just uncomfortable, it's a serious health issue that should be addressed. While typical remedies such as taking fiber supplements, eating prunes or consuming more water may help if one's diet is deficient, what is not so well understood is that having a daily routine that is out of tune with the natural cycles can also be a common cause of sluggish elimination. In addition to addressing any mental or emotional stress issues, which are often the primary cause of tense or dry bowels, a good tip for helping your friends and family become 'more regular' (of course you wouldn't get constipated yourself) is to get them to eat and sleep more in alignment with the daily cycles discussed here. Once this is done, assuming a reasonable diet is consumed, the need for even natural remedies for the symptomatic relief of sluggish bowels will usually disappear.

Happy bowels—Ideas to help

1. *Morning cleansing drink*

   As a general aid to assisting your body's natural inner cleansing and evacuation processes, start your day with a morning cleansing drink.

   First thing on arising each day, particularly if things are a little sluggish, drink the following:

   1 glass of ROOM TEMPERATURE WATER with
   10-20 drops of FRESH LEMON JUICE
   2-3 teaspoons of good quality ALOE VERA JUICE
   Females—do not include the aloe vera during the days of menstruation.

   * While fluids (water) taken first thing in the early morning should be at room temperature to assist bowel activity, Ayurveda generally recommends drinking warm or slightly hot water throughout the day.

2. *Toilet training*

   Another good habit to practice, especially if you tend to start moving before your bowels do in the morning, is to simply sit on the toilet for five or ten minutes. Don't read the morning paper, work out your day's 'to do' list or brainstorm your next novel. Just relax and have your attention on that part of your body. Directing your attention to any part of your body that is blocked or experiencing discomfort stimulates the natural intelligence to flow in that area and helps re-enliven its proper functioning.

   NOTE: In the case of severe constipation, it is important to avoid excessively straining or forcing things to arrive before they are ready. Regularly straining can aggravate or even create problems such as diverticulosis, haemorrhoids and hernias. It can also make your face look like it's impersonating a beetroot, which is not a good look!

The ancient art of squatting ... not sitting

As a quick side-note on the subject of dysfunctional bowels and constipation, it is interesting to highlight another area of natural wisdom in respect of our toilet habits. Many people from traditional Eastern cultures tell us that another reason we experience so many bowel-related problems in the West is our modern method of going to the toilet. Compared to the squatting method used by our ancestors and many Eastern cultures, we see our invention of toilet seats as an impressive sign of innovation, progress and being 'more civilized'. Unfortunately, while it may seem more comfortable, it is generally not healthy or conducive to the efficient elimination of our waste products. Anatomically, when we sit down on our haunches (i.e. squat), we naturally compress our intestines and encourage the efficient movement of bowel matter. Furthermore, the channel leading out the back door is positioned directly downward, thus taking advantage of gravity to assist smooth, force-free and problem-free evacuation. Western toilets put our bodies in a position that discourages this natural elimination. In the sitting position, faeces cannot travel through the bowels as freely. This can result in stagnation through to constipation.

While I don't expect too many people are going to rush out to demolish their toilet in preference to squatting over a hole in the floor (and fair enough), a more practical solution can be to simply have something to raise your feet and legs somewhat. Anything that you can conveniently fit in your bathroom which helps bring your thighs up to compress your abdominal area will provide good results. My mum, who will be infinitely pleased that I am telling the world about her bathroom habits, uses a 6-pack of toilet rolls. You could also use a small box or a 'stool'... pardon the pun! Another option is to simply lift your feet up and tuck your knees in or, alternatively, squat on the floor until '*showtime*'. When the participants are about to '*enter the arena*', simply sit on the toilet as normal. Of course, you could do as some of our smaller, lighter and more agile Asian and Middle Eastern friends have done since coming to the West. Many of them actually squat on the toilet seat itself. However, hearing of one gent being admitted to hospital with a piece of toilet seat in his you-know-what, I don't necessarily recommend this one!!!

Now, where were we?

Early morning exercise—the ideal daily kickstart

Aside from morningitis, you may have noticed the slower, heavier feel to the start of each new day. While we may not think of the slow, heavy, earthy qualities of nature as being positive ones necessarily, they are a perfect part of Mother Nature's rhythms. However, just because these qualities predominate in our body and our environment at this time doesn't mean we necessarily need to feel dull or sluggish. In addition to arising early, we can offset this tendency as Mother Nature intended us to—through activity.

In Ayurveda, the morning hours—around 6am to 8am—are recommended as the ideal time to exercise. Some activity at this time directly counteracts any heaviness or sluggishness we might otherwise experience, helps move the bowels should they need a little assistance, and stimulates metabolism, which is generally slower after a night's sleep. This is even more important for individuals with naturally slower and heavier constitutions. Without some activity to off set the earthy qualities predominating at this time, they may well feel congested, lethargic, and find it difficult to lose weight.

Regardless of the theory, our own experience confirms that we just feel so much better for the whole day when we start it with some exercise. In cultures with long histories of robust health, yoga or physical meditation-type activities have been routinely performed as a way of starting off the new day. Even today, as the sun rises around the world, thousands of people will perform Tai Chi in China, Zen-type practices in Japan and Surya Namaskar (the Salute to the Sun) on the banks of the Ganges in India.

According to our body's natural cycles, early morning exercise is the perfect way to start the day.

When practicalities prevent you from doing a significant amount of exercise in the morning, just do something light to get your body moving, such as a short walk, five minutes on an exercise bike, some stretching, home yoga or pilates.

Breakfast—'not' the most important meal of the day

The final activity to consider before heading off into the new day is breakfast.

If you have heard anything about healthy eating in recent times, you will no doubt be aware of the suggestion that 'breakfast is the most important meal of the day'. Alternatively, 'You need to have a good, hearty breakfast to get your day off on the right note'. Or, 'Eat breakfast like a king, lunch like a prince, dinner like a pauper'.

As this is a fairly universally accepted part of modern health science these days, it is worth seeing if it is true in terms of our natural cycles. Just as the early morning sun is relatively weak in strength, our digestive fire, which we need to digest food, is relatively weak in the early hours of the day. As such, most of us do not have strong appetites or the digestive strength to process much food at this time. Unlike modern health directives, in Ayurveda and other time-tested natural health sciences, breakfast is *not* recommended to be a large meal, let alone the most substantial meal of the day. In long-living groups such as the Okinawans, Vilcabambans, Campodimelani and Abkhasians, none have breakfast as the most important or substantial meal of the day. They have understood that the time when the sun reaches its peak is when we are best equipped to eat more.

Like all popular health recommendations, it is valuable first to understand why this tremendous focus on the importance of breakfast has come about. There are two main reasons.

i) One is our almost exclusive focus on weight loss and thus ways to stimulate metabolism, as opposed to an understanding of digestion and the cycles of digestion. Breakfast has been given relatively more 'importance', because eating food stimulates our metabolism and counters our body's calorie restriction response. This is particularly pertinent for people wanting to lose weight as metabolism is usually slower in the early morning hours and the body's natural inclination is to conserve calories if food is restricted, i.e. if one were to skip breakfast.

ii) Secondly, due to our hectic modern lifestyles and variable work shifts, taking the time to eat our main meal at lunch has largely gone the way of the dinosaur. As many people can go all day without a decent meal, eating a good breakfast has come to be seen as extremely important. This is not necessarily a bad thing in the circumstances, but it is good to appreciate that this is based on our current modern lifestyles and not on the natural cycles for peak health.

The modern wisdom surrounding breakfast is based largely on metabolism. Metabolism relates to the conversion of food by-products into energy within the cells of our body. However, before metabolism begins, we first need to digest the food we eat. By eating when our digestive strength tends to be weak, i.e. in the early morning, we are less likely to process our food properly. Poorly digested food is more likely to accumulate in our tissues and disturb the subtle flow of intelligence that runs our body. This is far more detrimental to long-term weight management and overall health than simply having a slow metabolism. Eating breakfast merely to stimulate metabolism or because we aren't going to eat properly until dinnertime is not the most enlightened way to good health.

Rather than eating breakfast to stimulate metabolism or because the diet plan says so, ancient natural wisdom suggests that we should eat breakfast based on whether we actually need food at this time, i.e. whether we are hungry!

(There's a novel idea—of course it may not be 'scientific' enough for some!)

From the Ayurvedic understanding, in addition to providing us with some energy to start the day, the purpose of breakfast is to '*kindle*' the digestive fire. Just as we put small twigs on a small fire in order to kindle the fire and make it strong, when breakfast is a relatively smaller, lighter meal, it stimulates or kindles our digestive fire. This helps it become strong and ready to digest our main meal at lunchtime. With thousands of years of collective wisdom behind them, in many traditional Asian and European cultures where obesity, diabetes and lethargy are largely non-existent, people have not eaten much if at all in the early morning hours. Throughout India, for example, many people would only consume cleansing-type drinks on arising. At about 10am, when the inner fire begins to rise in strength (like the sun), they would then take a short break and eat something light. In Hunza (northern Pakistan), researchers have studied the long-living and disease-defying inhabitants for decades and have found cancers, heart disease, diabetes and digestive conditions to be relatively rare occurrences. While there are a number of other factors that account for their longevity, it is rare for them to eat anything within a couple of hours of rising. Unlike in the West, where we think we have to eat first to get the energy to work, they work first and build up a strong appetite before taking their first food of the day.[b]

Once our natural digestive cycles are understood by people, many comment, 'That's funny because I'm usually not even hungry early in

---

b   As an interesting side-note, unlike the predominantly sweet breakfasts we eat in the West, which tend to dampen the digestive fire, even today many people from India, the Middle East and other parts of the world eat savory foods in the morning. Savory foods are known to stimulate the appetite.

the morning. I only eat because everyone says we should'. Often those on weight loss programs with structured and sometimes robotic menu plans, say, 'I'm suppose to have x, y or z for breakfast, but I just don't have the appetite for eating first thing in the morning'.

If you are trying to lose weight, naturally have a sluggish digestion or are simply not hungry in the mornings, don't eat just because you think you should. If possible, sip mildly hot water and drink warm juices on rising and eat a small, healthy snack, like fruit or wholemeal toast, if you are hungry around 10am. While practicalities prevent many of us from eating at this time, it is important to appreciate that our digestive fire will not be at its strongest at 6.30, 7.00 or 7.30am. Of course, if you have a strong appetite, by all means eat a decent breakfast. Athletes, laborers or those with naturally high metabolisms may well need a more substantial breakfast to satisfy their energy demands. But most of us do not. Listen to your body and don't be scared to follow the long-forgotten wisdom of common sense. If your body needs a hearty breakfast, it will tell you.

> The best way to determine how much breakfast to eat (apart from your actual hunger levels at the time) is according to your lunch-time appetite.
>
> If you are regularly hungry or low on energy by 11am, then obviously eat more at breakfast. However, if you get to 12.30 or 1pm without feeling genuinely hungry, cut down the amount you eat at breakfast.

* Many low carb diets, including the Atkins Diet, advocate hearty breakfasts such as bacon and eggs. These are certainly good 'hearty' breakfasts... good for a *'hearty attack'*!

THE LUNCHTIME CYCLE (10.00AM–2.00PM)—TIME TO EAT AND GET SOME SUN!

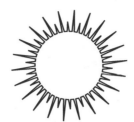

If you have ever been to Asia or Europe, you may have noticed, in more traditional places at least, that everything pretty well shuts down at lunchtime. In places like France or Italy, come lunchtime, if you aren't running a restaurant or café, you're sitting in one. Both historically and conventionally, there is a very good reason for this. The four-hour window between 10am and 2pm each day is known to be dominated by the qualities of fire and heat (Pitta). At this time of day, the sun or universal fire is at the peak of its power. Similarly, our body's central fire, our digestive fire, is also at the peak of its power. This is when we are maximally equipped physiologically to eat our main meal of the day. Just as we only put large logs on a fire once it is burning strongly, larger meals and heavier, hard-to-digest foods are best eaten in the middle of the day when we have the digestive strength to process them.

In ancient times, it was understood that eating our main meal at lunchtime brings many benefits:

1. As this is when our body's internal fire is naturally at its strongest, eating at this time gives us the opportunity to digest heavier foods and thus build strong disease-resistant tissues as well as deriving maximum energy and vitality.

2. Eating a healthy lunch is one of the best protections against wanting to binge eat or need a sugar fix later in the afternoon.

3. It is one of the best safeguards, along with a healthy afternoon tea, against hunger pangs and the tendency to overeat at night when digestion is weaker.

4. It helps align our body's other physiological functions, so that everything works optimally at their naturally designed times, e.g. the proper elimination of wastes. When one cycle is balanced and on time, all other internal cycles are more likely to be balanced and on time.

5. This is simply how our bodies have been designed for optimal health. It is also what the world's healthiest, metabolize populations have generally structured their daily routines around.

'Doesn't eating a big lunch mean a big sleep afterwards?'

If you are like most people considering the idea of eating your main meal at lunchtime, you may be thinking, 'If I eat a big meal at lunch, I will feel heavy and want to go to sleep. So how can that be?'

The best answer to this is given through an analogy. If you go to the petrol station to fill up your high performance car with fuel and not long after it konks out, there must generally be one of two problems. There is something wrong with the fuel that you put in your car, or there is something wrong with its engine. The same applies with our own high performance vehicles, our bodies. If you put food into your body at lunchtime and before long you start falling asleep, there is either something wrong with the quality of food you have eaten—your fuel—or there is a problem with your digestion—your engine.[10]

While some modern theorists say that eating carbohydrate-rich foods rather than protein-rich foods can also cause this problem, this generally has more to do with the consumption of largely refined carbohydrates. Refined carbohydrates tend to spike and then quickly drop our blood sugars. Carbohydrates are by nature energy-increasing. While starchy carbohydrates, such as pasta, can promote sleepiness more than protein-rich foods, when eaten in their unprocessed, natural state, in proper quantity and with a healthy digestion, such foods should be energy-promoting. Also, although it is suggested that lunch is ideally our main meal, this does not necessarily imply that it should be a 'big' meal. If we eat beyond our body's capacity to digest our food properly, even at lunchtime, we will experience heaviness, sluggishness and even sleepiness. The key, as always, is to listen to your body and honor your appetite rather than blindly eating what the diet plan says or whatever is on your plate.

> Reconnect yourself with the wisdom of ancient cultures and eat according to the cycle of the sun.
>
> When the sun is low, eat less. When the sun is high, eat more.

Lunchtime health—Ideas to help

1. If you do not already do so, then gradually begin making lunch your main meal of the day wherever possible. Give yourself a minimum of 30 minutes and preferably 45 minutes.

2. If you know in advance that you won't be able to eat at all around 12.30 or 1.00pm, look to eat earlier, e.g. 11.30am. This is still well within the four-hour peak digestion window and is much better than throwing something down on the run or not eating at all until much later in the day.

3. Alternatively, where it is genuinely impossible to have your main meal right in the middle of the day, just eat lightly at this time and then have another small meal, whenever convenient, later in the afternoon.

4. If you eat heavy, harder-to-digest foods such as meat, nuts, cheese, cheese sauces, raw salads or desserts, generally eat them at lunchtime rather than at dinnertime. (See Table 1 on page 79 for more on heavy and light foods.)

5. Don't confuse having your main meal of the day with having to eat a huge, all-you-can-eat feast. Whenever you eat, only eat according to your appetite.

6. Get some sun. The middle of the day is a critical time for going outside for some direct sunlight exposure. Despite popular recommendations to avoid the midday sun, some sunlight exposure at this time is absolutely vital for our health. (See the sunlight section in Wisdom Five for full details.)

Note for bosses:

If you are an employer, one of the best things you can ever do for your employees is to give them a decent lunchbreak. Long-term improvements in workers' productivity and performance from being able to eat properly and get some sun (brain) stimulation at lunchtime far outweigh any short-term losses. Less than 30 minutes for lunch should be considered a violation of workers' rights. It is certainly a violation of the natural cycles.

THE AFTERNOON CYCLE (2PM–6PM)—SIESTAS, AFTERNOON TEA & MANAGING THE ENERGY LOW

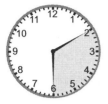

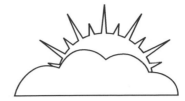

In Ayurveda, the period from 2pm to 6pm is known to be dominated by the qualities of space and air (Vata). As such, the qualities that are dominant in the environment and our bodies are by nature lighter, more airy, quick and changeable. This period can promote good bursts of creative activity, but can also make us more susceptible to sudden drops in energy, variable concentration and attention lapses. Modern science tells us that the post-lunch period corresponds to a significant drop in our blood sugars, and statistics from hospital admissions and car accidents suggest we are more likely to make mistakes at this time.

Right in the middle of this cycle, around 3–4pm, there are two common experiences. First, a mid-afternoon energy slump, with a corresponding desire for either a nana nap or a caffeine hit and second, a strong desire for something sweet. This is often known as a raid on the cookie jar, the cake shop or the chocolate bar stocks. While feeling tired or craving unhealthy sweets in the mid-afternoon is more indicative of a state of imbalance than balance, it is good to appreciate that there is some biological basis for such experiences at this time.

Siesta time

Throughout the ages, there have been two common ways of counteracting the natural afternoon energy low. Firstly, a short period of rest and secondly, having grounding, energy-promoting, sweet-tasting foods and beverages. When we think of big, traditional European lunches, we often think of the famous post-lunch 'siesta'. As siestas have been used in certain cultures for thousands of years, it begs the following questions. Is this idea of a siesta a good thing? Is it ideally a part of our natural daily cycles?

The general principle of a siesta, or grandpa nap, in the middle of the afternoon is a good one, particularly for those who are in the latter period of their lives—their wisdom years. Although in recent times the siesta has sometimes become regarded as more of an after-lunch practice (which can still have benefits), historically and physiologically, siestas are ideally taken in the mid-afternoon. In terms of the natural daily cycles, a short nana nap or the more dynamic sounding *'power nap'* is best around 3.30—4.30pm. This is when it most directly balances our natural energy low. However, it is important to note that having a siesta or mini-nap during the day, should only be done in a sitting or semi-reclined position. Ayurveda clearly states that day sleep, where one is lying in a horizontal position, closes down the subtle channels of the body (known as 'srotas'), tending to leave one duller and more sluggish.

The afternoon energy low should not be seen as a bad thing. You may remember having a mid-afternoon grandpa nap on weekends or holidays and feeling so much better for it. This is because it is actually Mother Nature's way of helping us re-energize and recharge. If we take a brief siesta or power nap at this time, we will likely bounce back with heightened energy and a higher level of performance, a *second wind*. It's like a rubber band. Only by pulling it back momentarily can it spring forward with increased power. Unfortunately, our busy lifestyles don't generally lend themselves to indulging in such luxuries. Instead, we commonly go for a caffeine hit, an energy drink or a sugary soft drink to get us through this energy lull. Such artificial stimulants can prop us up in the short term and give us a burst of energy and alertness, however they override what our body naturally wants to do, i.e. to recharge its batteries. Our rubber band cannot spring forward with renewed energy because it has not been pulled back. We eliminate our natural second wind and our energy levels come crashing back down once the caffeine or sugar hit has worn off. Worse, however, is that this whole process tends to throw out our natural energy cycle. This can reduce our energy levels at other times of the day and compromise our ability to fall asleep easily come bedtime. If you have any trouble getting to sleep at night, one of the first things to do is to eliminate any mid-afternoon stimulants and where possible take a mini break, do a short meditation or have some chillout time.

It is interesting to note that many famous high performers, including Leonardo da Vinci, Thomas Edison, Abraham Lincoln and Bill Clinton, were known to be regular catnappers. Modern research is also showing the tremendous benefits to our health and productivity from short power naps taken during the day. Benefits include increased alertness and cognitive function, reduced stress-related conditions and decreased reliance on stimulants such as coffee or other caffeine products.[11] In the corporate world, mini breaks and even power naps are increasingly being promoted within the workplace as a way of reducing burnout and boosting productivity. Some workplaces now even invest in *sleep pods*, which are specially designed capsules that allow and promote power naps in office environments. As common convention associates napping with laziness or reduced performance, this is most interesting! Very soon, napping in the afternoon will once again be seen as a key to peak performance, health and productivity. We will again reinvent the wheel that our 'less progressive' ancestors knew about thousands of years ago, and then herald it as another groundbreaking new discovery of modern science.

A mid-afternoon siesta or power nap can be a marvelous boon for long-term health.

While usually not practical or imperative within a busy Western lifestyle, if you are retired, elderly, work more than ten hours a day, or are simply able to take a short rest in the afternoon, by all means do so.

Afternoon tea

In addition to a short period of rest, the other way to balance the afternoon energy low is through healthy energy-boosting foods and drinks. The consumption of refreshing, energizing, sweet-tasting foods and drinks in the mid to late afternoon has been an integral part of many traditional cultures' routines for millennia. Drinks have included coconut juice in the tropics, sweet lassi in India and herbal tea throughout Japan and China. Sweet foods and drinks are earthier by nature and thus provide a practical means of settling our active minds and grounding our restless bodies. It is vitally important to balance our mind and body at this time. If we don't, the space and air qualities that predominate can easily become excessive. Instead of feeling grounded, we can feel 'spacey' or 'airy'. This can create further problems later in the evening when we can't stop ourselves from overeating at dinnertime (our way of trying to ground ourselves), or prevent our busy minds from spacing out and so impairing our ability to get to sleep.

Good options for afternoon tea include sweet juicy fruits, nuts, minimally processed energy bars and sweet drinks, depending on the season. In spring and summer, coconut, pineapple and apple juices can be great. In winter, sweet teas may be preferred. Some cultures drink tea all year round, but simply vary what type of tea depending on the season, for instance warming ginger or clove-based teas in winter and cooling rose petal or mint teas in summer. While high intakes of refined sugary items are obviously not ideal at any time, if you do have an as yet uncontrollable sweet tooth and need a sweet treat such as a cake, biscuit or chocolate, then afternoon tea is as good a time as any to indulge. At least at this time, rather than at night, your body is better able to process these heavier, harder-to-digest foods while your digestion is stronger.

Second chance exercise

Where early morning exercise is not practical, the next best time for some physical activity according to the natural cycles is in this late afternoon or early evening period. As physical activity stimulates both our metabolism and our nervous system, exercising well into the evening can interfere with our body's natural desire to wind down after dark. Two of the most common times people exercise today, which directly violate our body's natural cycles, are at lunchtime and beyond the early part of the evening cycle. Go into any centrally located gymnasium at 7, 8 or even 9 o'clock at night and you will see dozens of people huffing and puffing their way to health and fitness. While such desire and commitment to exercise is fantastic and benefits will certainly be derived, activity at this time, particularly strenuous exercise, interferes with what our bodies naturally want to do, i.e. slow down in readiness for optimal sleep. Although vigorous exercise in the middle of the day is also not ideal (it's better to be eating and digesting our main meal), it is the only practical time that some people have to do it and can be done with relatively few consequences. However, this is not the case with regular nighttime activity.

> Regularly exercising late into the evening directly opposes our body's natural desire to slow down its metabolic activity in preparation for optimal sleep.
>
> While the practicalities of fitting everything into our busy Western lives can be difficult, if you like or need to exercise later in the day, try finishing by around 7 or 7.30pm most nights.

The following diagram summarizes the activities that are most in tune with the body's natural daily cycles.

Diagram 2: The Daily Clock

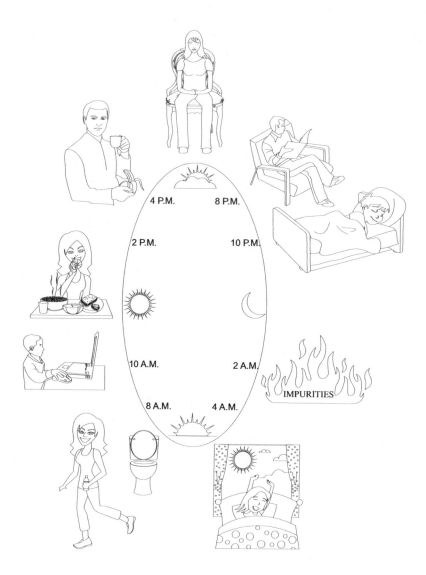

Morning
Arise early (with the birds)
Evacuate the bowels
Meditation / Sun gazing *
Exercise or brief physical activity
Light breakfast

Lunchtime
Main meal of the day
Sunlight exposure where possible

Mid-afternoon
Short siesta / power nap (optional)
Natural, energy-boosting foods and drinks

Late afternoon
Meditation
Exercise or activity
Sun gazing (optional) *

Evening
Eat light
Mentally relaxing activities
Bed early (10—10.30pm or earlier) most nights

Night
Sleep **

* Sun gazing is discussed in Wisdom Five
** If at any time you can't remember what the ideal daily cycles are,
just observe most modern-day teenagers ... and do the exact opposite!

Seed wisdom

In Mother Nature's world, and according to the eternal laws of health, *'timing is everything'*. It's not just what we do, but when we do it.

One of the most marked differences between healthy, disease-resistant cultures and our own high-stress, high-disease society is our growing violation of the natural daily cycles. Traditional cultures haven't had You Tube, late-night TV or 10pm happy hour to tempt them away from their natural cycles. As such, most of them have generally eaten their main meal during the day, eaten lightly at night and gone to bed soon after the setting of the sun. In contrast, we have progressively begun diminishing the importance of lunch, eating our main meals after dark (when we have little digestive capacity), and going to bed later and later.

The more we can align our lives with the eternal rhythms of Mother Nature, the more our bodies will enjoy good energy, vitality, quality sleep, healthy weight and overall good health.

Live in tune with Mother Nature's daily cycles.

Wisdom Three

Eat 'Intelligent' Food

Did you ever stop to taste a carrot?
Not just eat it, but taste it? You can't taste the
beauty and energy of the earth in a Twinkie.
Astrid Alauda

Just take a moment to listen to your body.

What do I mean, *listen* to your body?

We think of our bodies as concrete, physical structures. However, from the understanding of both the most highly developed cultures throughout history and the latest discoveries of quantum physics, at the basis of everything in our universe, including our bodies, is nothing other than energy or sound. At their deepest level, our bodies are nothing other than intelligence. This intelligence manifests into different sounds, or energetic vibrations, that become the subatomic particles, atoms, cells, tissues, organs and organ systems of our physical bodies. It is said that if we were able to raise our level of consciousness to that of an enlightened sage, we could literally hear the sounds at the basis of our own minds and bodies. The sages suggest that, like the individual musicians in an orchestra, each of our body's organs or tissues has its own distinct vibration or individual resonance. As a gross hypothetical example, our livers might go 'ding ding ding', our kidneys might go 'bing bing bing' and our brainstems might go 'ting ting ting'. Although each body part has its own signature sound, holistically our bodies are like a symphony. This is the music, or 'vibrational sound', of optimal health. When in tune, all our physiological functions flow more easily and the communication between our cells is unrestricted and health-promoting. Conversely, ill health results when our internal musicians (our cells and tissues) lose their natural melody or get out of resonance with each other. Instead of the liver going 'ding ding ding', it might start to sound like 'doong doong doong'.

Interestingly, the way time-tested natural health sciences suggest we maintain or restore health on the gross level of our cells or tissues is not to target them directly. A more effective means is to alter the underlying music or vibrational field. This is similar to the old science experiment where you put dozens of iron filings on a piece of paper and hold a small magnet beneath the paper. By simply changing the magnet's position slightly, you can create a completely new pattern of the filings on top of the paper. In essence, by affecting the underlying intelligence or vibration (that which we can't see), we create profound changes on the surface level of life. The same is true for our bodies. The ancients suggest that in any moment of our existence we can create a whole new body for ourselves, simply by changing the underlying vibrations that manifest into our cells and tissues.

Now what's all this got to do with food? The answer is absolutely everything.

In Part I we discussed how we are intimately connected to the natural world around us. The intelligence that runs our bodies runs all of life.

In traditional medical sciences such as Ayurveda and Tibetan medicine, just like our bodies, food at its basis was seen to be nothing other than packets of intelligence. Different foods were understood to have their own unique sound vibration, or frequency, just as our different organs and tissues do. In this light, when we think of our plant kingdom, we can see that it has its own orchestra, made up of an infinitely diverse range of fruits, vegetables, beans, nuts, grains and various other players. If you've ever been in a forest and closed your eyes, in the silence you may have heard the pulsating sounds of Mother Nature's orchestra. When we eat foods that are alive with Mother Nature's intelligence, we take in the different sound vibrations that strengthen the various cells, tissues and organs of our bodies. Like a musician re-tuning their violin, we re-tune and recalibrate our bodies by eating these foods.

Up until now, you may have thought of eating food as merely filling your stomach and providing some nourishment in the form of carbohydrates, fats and vitamins. However, as understood by our wisest ancestors, there is a far deeper wisdom: the true purpose of eating is to imbibe intelligence. It is the intrinsic intelligence found in natural foods that enables these foods to properly direct and utilize their basic nutrients. Simply focusing on fats, carbohydrates or vitamins, without imbibing the intelligence by which to activate and organize them, is like getting a group of classical musicians together without a conductor. We might get some nice individual notes and melodies, but there will be no synergy, no harmony ... no beautiful music. Only by eating foods that are alive with intelligence can we promote our highest level of health.

> The highest wisdom of nutrition lies well beyond fats, carbohydrates and calories.
>
> It lies in the field of food 'intelligence.'
>
> It is a food's unique vibrational resonance and holistic intelligence that truly make the various cells and tissues of our bodies dance with health.

Intelligent and non-intelligent foods

Think of the intelligence of nature at work in growing a fruit tree. The exquisite intelligence of life is fully alive in the fruit of that tree. You take a beautifully ripe apple, orange or mango and bite into it. Instantaneously, you get a burst of its intelligence resonating within you. It's *alive*. It feels good. It doesn't just taste good—it resonates with your whole body. The same applies if you were to eat freshly grown vegetables straight from a garden. Think of driving through the country and seeing the fields of golden wheat springing up from the ground—nature at its best. Add some sun, some water and connection to the earth itself, and you have the perfect recipe, beautifully put together by the wisest Master Chef herself, Mother Nature. These are examples of intelligent foods.

Now think about the last time you ate fruit out of a plastic container. How does it compare? Think about the old, processed cereals with artificially manipulated milk and highly refined sugar that many of us have for breakfast. Hmmm. What about the canned spaghetti, zapped in the microwave and eaten on refined white bread with laboratory-made margarine, or the three-day-old reheated meals made from packaged vegetables we had for dinner? From the perspective of modern science, all these things may have some nutritional value. Read the side of the tin or package—your first clue as to how much natural intelligence a food has—and you can read all about the carbohydrates, proteins, vitamins and minerals. It all sounds good, but unfortunately there is nothing indicating how much intelligence there is in the food. Actually, I should have said 'fortunately' because with all the above examples, as with any food that is old or highly processed, there is rarely any intelligence left. Most breakfast cereals are so highly processed that there is more nutrition in the cardboard boxes they come in! The health-promoting vibrations of the original natural foods they come from are left at the food processing plant long before we get to eat them.

All such foods can be considered non-intelligent or 'intelligence-extracted' foods. When we consume foods that lack intelligence, we take in vibrations incongruent with our body's internal orchestra and significantly compromise the intelligent functioning of our cells. Over time our bodies become *out of tune*. They lose their natural harmony and sense of ease. Lack of cellular harmony and ease is what ancient medicine men and women have said expresses itself initially as lack of energy, fatigue and mental dullness, and eventually as 'dis-harmony' and 'dis-ease'.

Three keys to intelligent foods

From the understanding of the natural sciences, we can isolate three key principles of intelligent, natural foods. We will look at each in detail.

INTELLIGENT FOOD KEY 1—WHOLE FOODS

In all the decades of research on the healthiest, metabolize peoples of our world, no finding has been as universal or as well-documented as the fact that they have subsisted almost entirely on natural, 'whole foods'.

Common to the Hunzans, Vilcabambans, Abkhasians, Campo-dimelani, Symiots and other age-defying groups has been a close connection to locally grown, natural, whole food produce. Whole foods are simply foods that haven't had any vital parts of the food extracted. Whole foods are easy to find. They are simply Mother Nature's foods, such as naturally grown fruits, vegetables, nuts, seeds and grains. By eating foods whole, the intrinsic intelligence and the incomprehensible synergies of all the diverse plant parts, as developed by Mother Nature over millennia, are fully retained. This ensures that the so-called 'active ingredients' get to the cellular destinations they need to, while creating side benefits and not side effects.

Although fats have been on the receiving end of some bad publicity in recent times, for millennia indigenous cultures have known that fats found in whole foods such as avocadoes, seeds and nuts are wholly healthy. Even if we eat too much of them, our bodies can recognize, process and eliminate these types of fats without harm, provided that our level of consumption does not compromise our ability to digest them. Carbohydrates too are now often the subject of much bad press. However, carbohydrates in Mother Nature's whole foods are also completely healthy. You will never put on weight eating moderate amounts of high carbohydrate foods when they are in whole food form. The whole debate (pardon the pun) about good and bad fats, or good and bad carbohydrates, is simply based on ignorance. This is what those who profit from our ignorance want. If you remain ignorant, they will convince you that totally unnatural and often health-compromising low fat and low carb foods are healthy. Keep it simple. Bad fats and bad carbohydrates are simply those made in scientific laboratories. Natural, whole foods, even those that are high in fats or carbohydrates, contain vibrational energies that will nourish, strengthen and enliven every area of your body.

> In terms of nutrition, what is most important is what form our food is in and whether it retains its holistic intelligence.
>
> It is a food's intelligence that determines what our bodies do with it once we've eaten it.

Food signatures—the ultimate example of Mother Nature's whole food intelligence

The Gods created certain kinds of beings to replenish our bodies, they are the trees and the plants and the seeds.

Plato

As discussed, most traditional medical sciences understood that foods, like our bodies, are literally 'packets of intelligence', each with its own unique sound vibration or frequency. However, this wasn't just a general concept, the specific vibrational effects of different foods were known in exquisite detail. This was achieved through the understanding that Mother Nature uses the same 'patterns of intelligence' whether she is creating DNA, a cell, a tree, a flower, a human body, or even an entire universe. The patterns are all the same. In Ayurveda, these correlations are known through the 'Law of Similarities'. They have also been understood through the 'Hermetic Law of Correspondence' and the 'Doctrine of Signatures'—*that which is like unto* itself is drawn'. The Doctrine of Signatures details how the color, shape and texture of different whole foods tell us what parts of our bodies these foods specifically nourish. Thanks to Don Tolman[1], one of the world's leading whole foods teachers, the ancient knowledge of food signs has recently been re-enlivened through many of his fascinating correlations with modern-day science. These correlations further demonstrate how the foods we eat have a far greater holistic purpose than merely supplying nutrient x, y or z.

2800 years ago, the ancient Greeks noticed that walnuts looked just like the human brain. Through the ancient science of observation, they saw that walnuts had distinct left and right hemispheres, wrinkles or folds just like our brain's cerebral cortex, and were even contained in a hard shell just like our skull. Science now tells us that when eaten, a walnut's active ingredients are able to cross our important blood-brain barrier and stimulate the production of important neurotransmitters, including serotonin, for optimal brain function. The oil in walnuts is also known to help break down plaque build-ups in our brain. Walnuts don't just look like brains and provide nutrients such as healthy fatty acids, they specifically nourish our brain, memory and mental function.

Carrots, when cut, look just like the iris and pupil of an eye. Carrots don't simply provide beta-carotene, traditionally they were known to nourish the eyes in an energetic and vibrational sense.[a] Beetroots, which look just like red blood cells, don't simply provide iron, they are known to specifically nourish our blood. Celery stalks aren't just long and slen-

---

a   Modern science is split on whether carrots are good for eyesight. This is in part due to the fact that science tends to focus on individual nutrients such as beta-carotene or vitamin A, rather than the holistic vibrational resonance eff ects of the whole food. The same applies for other foods.

der like human bones; celery also contains a similar percentage of bone-strengthening nutrients, such as sodium, to that found in human bones. Sweet potatoes don't just resemble the pancreas. Despite their name, sweet potatoes are known to help balance blood sugars just like insulin, which is released from the pancreas. Thousands of years ago, American Indians noticed that a tomato and a human heart both possess a similar shape, color and unique four hollow chamber design. Many nutritionists today suggest that tomatoes are good for the heart.

Last but not least is the avocado. Avocadoes, when cut lengthwise into two halves, look like either a female womb and cervix or a pregnant female (the half with the seed intact). Avocadoes do far more than just supply some vitamin E or potassium. They were known traditionally to target the female organs of reproduction. This is why in ancient times the Mayans and Incas used to offer avocadoes to pregnant women as a gift to mother and baby. Interestingly, today's science now suggests that avocadoes can help reduce cervical cancers, balance female hormones during pregnancy, and reduce unwanted birth weight after pregnancy. And how long does Mother Nature take to grow an avocado from blossom to ripened fruit? Nine months.

Male and female foods

According to Tolman, a further illustration of the inherent intelligence in whole foods is shown in the understanding of how different foods nourish men and women in different ways. While we are either male or female, according to ancient wisdom, each one of us is actually made up of both masculine and feminine qualities or energies. Similarly, all of Mother Nature's foods were known to possess a predominantly female or male intelligence. Female foods were seen to be sweeter, more intuitive and could multi-task, while male foods could only be eaten one at a time, needed more regular washing, and went off quickly if not attended to! Seriously, foods that physically resemble the typical female body shape, the traditional *pear shape,* were known to predominantly nourish the feminine energy and female organs. Such foods include avocadoes, eggplant and pears themselves. Foods such as oranges, grapefruits and other citrus fruits that look like female breasts are now known to assist the movement of lymph in and out of the breasts. Some modern research has also begun to show associations between citrus fruits and breast cancer protection.[2] Melons and coconuts, terms sometimes used derogatorily to describe female breasts due to their strong resemblance, were also known to nourish the breasts. In Ayurveda, coconut juice has long been considered par excellence for nourishing the female breast tissue, and similar juices are commonly prescribed for breast-feeding mothers, as they are known to directly nourish breast milk.

Conversely, foods resembling the primary male reproductive organ were believed to strengthen masculine energy (bananas, zucchinis, cucumbers) and stimulate male sexual energy (peanuts). Interestingly, arginine, an amino acid found in rich supply in peanuts, is today one of the main constituents of ... Viagra! Ladies, beware a certain someone emptying the peanut bowl at your next party! Kiwi fruits and fresh figs, which grow in pairs of two, both look like male testicles and are full of 'seeds'. Figs and kiwi fruits are thought to boost the motility, volume and health of sperm.

While from a modern scientific perspective any of these correlations may be deemed less than categorical, it is good to appreciate that the law of similarities works at a far deeper level of nature's wisdom than isolated nutritional components. It is the holistic effect of foods on the electrical energy pattern of the organs they target that delivers their ultimate nourishment. In this light, these examples and many more further point to the fundamental and unequivocal intelligence of Mother Nature's whole foods.

> Plant whole foods are like tuning forks for our body.
>
> The colors, shapes and textures of whole foods are literally Mother Nature's signs to us (i.e. signatures or 'signs of nature') of what parts of our body are balanced, strengthened and healed when we eat them.
>
> If your body needs a tune-up, eat the corresponding whole foods.

* One could ask, 'What if I don't know all the different food signatures?' Fortunately, we don't even need to know them in detail. Mother Nature always makes things simple. At a deep unconscious level, the fact that we find a certain fruit or vegetable's smell, shape, color or texture pleasing or desirable is a sign that it is balancing for us. If certain foods do not appeal, that can be a sign that our body may not need so much of that food at that time. Of course, this all depends on being in a state of relative balance. When we get stressed, our natural, intelligent desires for food can get distorted. If in doubt, just try to follow the signs.

Processed foods—sickness-promoting foods

If we're not willing to settle for junk living, we certainly shouldn't settle for junk food.

Sally Edwards

Appreciating the unseen intelligence present in natural, whole foods, we can now see why consuming even moderate quantities of modern, processed foods can unquestionably jeopardize our health.

Processed foods, by their very nature, are the exact opposite of high-intelligence foods. Processed foods have certain parts—and therefore certain vitamins, minerals and fibers—stripped away. Other valuable nutrients are lost in the manufacturing and storing process. Some vitamins, such as vitamin C, are heat sensitive, yet many modern-day processes use high heat. Then guess what happens? Vitamins and minerals get artificially added back into the food. Think of the cereal ads. 'Fortified with over half the recommended daily intake of vitamins C and E, B1, iron and folate! 'Fortified or enriched with' makes it sound as if you are getting something superior. Yet most of these nutrients, for example thiamine (vitamin B1) which helps release energy from carbohydrates, are actually removed in the refining process. Food manufacturers are just trying to prop up what they have previously taken out. First they destroy the holistic synergy of Mother Nature's foods, and then try to re-place them with artificial (unintelligent) substitutes. Most importantly, it is not just gross nutrition that gets taken out in processed foods but the unseen intelligence of the original whole food. To top things off , they add in some health-compromising chemical additives and preservatives and then run marketing campaigns to make you think that you are getting the heights of nutrition. Don't be fooled.

Western A. Price was one of the world's pioneering nutritional researchers. Over fifty years ago, he graphically illustrated the marked physical degeneration in individuals who changed from eating natural foods to regularly consuming unnatural, highly processed, Western foodstuffs.[3] A dentist by training, Price travelled throughout some of the most remote regions of the world. He studied the dietary habits of Scottish Highlanders, Australian Aborigines, the Maasai of Africa, Indigenous Canadian tribes, Alaskan Eskimos and many others. Despite a wide range of diets being consumed—ranging from fish-eating Eskimos, wild game-eating Amazonian hunter gatherers and dairy-eating Swiss villagers, to various cultures who predominantly existed on plant foods—Price found one common factor to be responsible for all these cultures' robust health. It was the fact that they ate natural, whole foods. In stark contrast to the children and adults who had consumed Western diets—with large amounts of refined sugars, processed foods and white flour—the incidence of tooth decay, narrowed faces, under-developed facial features or any other 'facial deformities' was almost non-existent in these cultures. Countering the argument that these differences were genetically or racially based, Price was able to document and show through pictures that such instances of physical deterioration came about when individuals gave up a traditional diet of natural whole foods in favor of modern, processed foods. These foods included refined sugars, refined grains such as white bread, pasteurized milks and processed vegetable oils.

Many of our world's indigenous cultures have slowly been introduced to highly processed Western diets in recent decades. Along with this trend, Price was able to show significant correlations, not only with dental deformities but also with other problems such as lowered immunity, a higher rate of birth defects and increased disease in both adults and children. Shockingly, the time for such deterioration to take place in those who diverted from a predominantly natural, whole food diet to what Price called '*devitalizing*' foods was often within one generation of a culture. Price specifically commented that indigenous cultures, including the Australian Aborigines who lived for thousands of years without any significant number of dental deformities, developed a high number of cases of serious deterioration the generation after they adopted the '*foods of the white man*'.[4] Up until the early 1900's, diabetes was basically unknown in many Aboriginal and Native American tribes. Now, as many of these groups move further and further from their traditional diets and consume more Western foods, the incidence of diabetes is skyrocketing. While there are undoubtedly many other associated factors involved in the decline of an indigenous population's health, the influence of processed foods is certainly one that we would do well to take heed of.

> If Mother Nature's whole foods are high-intelligence, health-creating foods, then highly processed foods can be seen as unintelligent (dumb), sickness-promoting foods.

The dangers of whole food destruction

The following are just a few examples of how modern-day food processing destroys the synergies in whole foods, thus disrupting their natural intelligence and compromising our health.

1. Homogenized milk

Homogenization is a mechanical process where milk in its natural state is forced through tiny holes under pressure of up to 2,500 psi. As the average pressure recommended for car tyres is about 34—40 psi, you get an idea of how natural this is! For what benefit to our health is this done? Well, none. It's done so that there is no unhealthy looking cream at the top of our milk, i.e. so that it 'looks nicer'. Although it might be more aesthetically pleasing, unfortunately no one bothered to ask our body cells what they thought of this process.

Homogenized milk becomes less stable to heat, more sensitive to oxidation, and the fat molecules get smashed to smithereens. Our body cells have evolved over millennia to break down and process fat molecules when the molecules are in their natural state (unhomogenized). This is largely done by our bile salts. When the fats are deformed by homogenization, however, our bile salts can't break down the fats properly. Being so small, the fats can pass through the gut wall without being 'digested' or broken down properly. Once these deformed fat molecules move into our body proper, they are not in a form that our body cells recognize. As such, even the elimination of these now health-compromising rather than health-promoting fats is disturbed.

When we destroy the natural state of fat molecules, or in the case of skim or low fat milks artificially remove most of the fat, we also remove the natural synergies that allow the proper absorption and assimilation of the fat and other nutrients. Many people drink milk for the calcium. However, by drinking processed varieties where the natural milk fats are damaged or missing, for example in homogenized or skim milks, we actually compromise our ability to absorb nutrients such as calcium. While there is some debate about this in scientific circles, when viewed from the understanding of the body's natural intelligence and interdependent synergies, it makes perfect sense. Everything in nature is interconnected. We know that when we destroy the parts, we compromise the whole, but it's also true that when we destroy the whole, we automatically compromise the parts.

2. Refined wheat—white flour

Wheat as created by Mother Nature is 'whole' wheat. It contains a fiber-rich bran (wheatbran), a nutrient-rich germ (wheatgerm) and an endosperm. All these were put in by Mother Nature for good reason. When combined, they are why ancient cultures throughout time have honored wheat for its nourishing, strengthening and health-promoting effects. Homemade, whole wheat breads have been a staple part of the diets of many of the world's metabolize cultural groups, including the Hunzans, Campodimelani and Symiots.

Because in the West we tend to be averse to anything that might actually promote our health, we process wheat by stripping off the germ and bran. In the process, we also strip most of its natural, health-promoting goodness. Why would we do this? The germ is removed because this helps increase the shelf life of products that contain wheat! Wheatgerm promotes our health and longevity, but who wants that when we can have our bread last longer? This stripping of vital parts of the grain is essentially the difference when we decide to eat white flours or white breads as opposed to whole wheat flours or wholegrain breads.

In most highly developed countries, over 95% of the wheat consumed is in its highly refined form. However, our body's inner intelligence has been developed over eons to recognize wheat in its natural form. Refined flour products, such as white bread, are not simply devoid of optimal nutrition, they lack the intelligence of natural wheat. Lacking their proper whole food resonance, they actually disturb our natural digestive process and can indirectly promote ill health over time. As has been said, 'the whiter the bread, the quicker you're dead'.[5]

* It is noted that a good percentage of our population these days has wheat and/or dairy allergies or intolerances. This is far more common than it used to be. I've never come across any literature that suggests any traditional cultures have had such widespread problems. While there are obviously genuine cases of wheat and dairy (lactose) allergies, in many cases it could reasonably be surmised that it is not actually the wheat or dairy that is at fault but rather the unnatural, modern ways in which we consume them. Ayurveda would add that having a less than optimally functioning digestive system, due to factors such as poor eating practices or high stress lifestyles, can also play a significant role in these problems.

3. Margarine

As for butter versus margarine, I trust cows more than chemists.

Joan Gussow

Today, food companies, many doctors and even some dieticians commonly recommend us to eat supposedly healthy margarine instead of evil butter. But should we listen to them?

As always, the first question to ask is, 'Are margarines or margarine spreads naturally occurring foods?' The answer is absolutely not. While starting out as a natural product, margarines are artificially manipulated and highly processed. Synthetic or isolated natural ingredients are added by food technologists for the purpose of trying to control specific aspects of health such as cholesterol. However, trying to control individual aspects of health in isolation is a recipe for disaster as our bodies work holistically. All parts are interrelated.

Adding health-promoting substances such as plant-based sterols to completely unnatural, laboratory-made products does not make them healthy. In fact, while plant sterols may help reduce cholesterol, they can also block the absorption of important fat soluble vitamins such as vitamin A and vitamin D.

Years ago, scientists felt the saturated fats in foods like butter were bad for our hearts, so they made polyunsaturated margarines as a supposedly healthier alternative. Unfortunately, these polyunsaturated fats were found to be easily oxidized and thus subjected us to far greater free radical damage. It is largely oxidative damage to cholesterol rather than just having high cholesterol that is associated with the harmful plaque-like substances linked to conditions such as heart disease. The problem was merely shifted not solved. The same is happening again. These days we know a lot more about the great harm done to people's health from trans fats. Trans fats have been extensively used in margarines until recently, and are still found in high quantities in products such as fried foods, breakfast bars and pastries. Trans fats are fats formed when liquid oils are turned into solid fats through hydrogenation—for example, when vegetable oils are hardened into margarine or shortening. These are called *'partially hydrogenated vegetable oils'* or PHVO's. PHVO's are seen as extremely dangerous because they raise our levels of the supposedly 'bad' cholesterol (LDL) and lower our levels of good cholesterol (HDL). They have also been closely associated with many serious diseases, particularly cardiovascular disease[6], stroke and type 2 diabetes. PHVO's are totally artificial and are manufactured for the express purpose of … wait for it … helping food manufacturers increase the shelf life of their products!

Dr Michael Jacobson, Executive Director of the US Center for Science in the Public Interest, says, 'Unlike fats that occur in nature, partially hydrogenated vegetable oil (PHVO) is totally artificial and absolutely unnecessary in the food supply'. In one of the all-time great quotes he wisely adds, 'Food processing companies should worry less about the shelf life of their products and more about the shelf life of their customers. Getting rid of PHVO is probably the single easiest, fastest, cheapest way to save tens of thousands of lives each year'.

Thanks to the tremendous work done by people like Dr Jacobson, we consumers—and food manufacturers—are now realizing the gross danger to our health that trans fats present. As a result, their inclusion in food is being reduced in most countries around the world. They are actually banned beyond minimal limits in countries like Denmark and Switzerland and must be labelled in the US. Unfortunately, at the time of writing, such restrictions are yet to be implemented in Australia.

Even today's so-called healthy margarines or margarine spreads, the ones without trans fats and with added 'cholesterol-lowering plant phenols', are not naturally occurring and should not be seen as healthy. Just take a look at the ingredients list and see all the synthetic anti-oxidants, thickeners, preservatives and colors that have been added!

So what should you do if you have high cholesterol? One suggestion would be to learn from the peoples of Hunza, Vilcabamba and Abkhasia as well as the millions of rural folk who have lived in countries like China and Japan. In such places, where a predominantly whole food, plantbased diet has been eaten, the problems of high cholesterol are basically... zero. That's nil. None. Zilch. High cholesterol is almost entirely a Western lifestyle phenomenon, strongly associated with stress and high intakes of animal foods. Although food manufacturers and drug companies don't want you to know this, lowering cholesterol is not difficult and can be done entirely naturally. How? By simply reducing stress levels, eating fewer animal products (particularly red meat) and consuming a predominantly plant-based, whole food diet. Plant foods not only contain zero cholesterol but also actively balance out high cholesterol. Instead of margarine, use things like avocado, minimally processed nut butters and extra virgin olive oil for spreads and dips. Natural wisdom suggests that we should not eat products manufactured in scientific laboratories to artificially reduce what is only 'high' because of a poor diet or lifestyle. Keep it simple. Eat natural foods.

4. Salt

Salt is born of the purest of parents—the sun and the sea.

Pythagoras

In the classic Western way of making things black and white—salad is good, fat is bad—salt has been put in the 'bad' camp. However, the ancients treasured salt and knew it was one of the most critical ingredients for a healthy body. Almost 5000 years ago, the Chinese pharmacological text, the *Peng-Tzao-Kan-Mu*, listed the medicinal effects of 40 varieties of natural salt.[7] In the ancient world, before money or gold, salt was used to represent trust and value. You might have been 'worth your salt' or considered the 'salt of the earth'. We are now paid a 'salary' which comes from the same word as salt. Roman soldiers used to be paid in salt because it was universally 'trusted' or relied upon. This was when people ate real salt. Real or 'good' salt contains 80 or more naturally occurring minerals and healing ingredients, other than sodium chloride, that are synergistically put together by Mother Nature. Way back before the time of ancient Rome and Greece, this type of salt was known to strengthen, balance and heal the body.

Good salt—salt that occurs naturally—plays a primary role in the proper functioning of the nervous system, helps maintain a healthy fluid balance in the body, and contributes to many important chemical reactions. Ancient healers considered good salt to be one of their most prized medicines. For thousands of years, salt was one of the first things used to heal infections and treat inflammation. Have you ever had a cut or skin rash that seemed to take forever to get better, but after swimming in the ocean a couple of times, it 'miraculously' healed? Good salt was also known to be absolutely critical to bone health. Do you know where coral, which forms large parts of tropical ocean floors, comes from? From calcium ions the corals acquire from seawater. The calcium comes from ionized sodium when sunlight shines through 'salt' water. A similar process occurs in our bodies. Sodium (salt) is first ionized into calcium, and then into the 100-plus other minerals that make up our body.[8] Good salt also helps cleanse the lining of the intestinal tract, improving the efficiency of digestion and absorption. Insufficient good, or naturally occurring salt, in one's diet can greatly impair overall mineral health, cause problems such as migraines or tension headaches, irritability, pain, lack of food satisfaction (and thus overeating), and contribute to weak bones and conditions such as osteoporosis.

So why does salt have such a bad name? The reason is that we eat too much 'rubbish' salt instead of real salt. Most of the current misunderstanding regarding salt stems from our modern-day processing of this wonder mineral (surprise surprise!). Nowadays, most commercial salts that we eat, e.g. highly processed regular table salt, have most of natural salt's 80-plus health-promoting minerals stripped away. (Food manufacturers consider them 'impurities'!) Even worse, regular, processed salts often have dangerous anti-caking agents like magnesium carbonate and aluminum silicate added in to make them flow better. This type of imposter salt is 'bad' salt. Eating this type of salt will certainly contribute to all the problems typically associated with salt.

Appreciate that the bad press surrounding salt is mainly due to the high consumption of fast or highly processed foods, and the overuse of refined, totally unnatural varieties of salt. Salt is not bad for you. In its naturally occurring state, in the right quantity, it is one of Mother Nature's most wonderful healing gifts and one of the most critical ingredients for your optimal health. Eat it, swim in it, bathe in it. Keep it natural and enjoy it.

5. Refined sugars

Sugar has certainly had its fair share of bad press in recent years. From rotting our teeth and spiking our blood sugars to containing 'empty calories', it's certainly not very high up on most people's Christmas list. However, have you ever wondered why Mother Nature covered so much of our planet with sugar cane if it was so bad for us?

From a natural wisdom perspective, small quantities of sugar can be seen as a perfectly healthy way of contributing the essential sweet taste to our overall diet. In Ayurveda, the sweet taste is one of six essential tastes in our diet—the others being sour, salty, pungent, bitter and astringent. The sweet taste is considered vital to both our emotional and general health and ideally comes from sweet foods such as wheat, rice, dairy or sweet fruits and vegetables. With the exception of pre-existing conditions such as diabetes or cancer, in its natural, untampered state, 'small' quantities of sugar can be considered a perfectly healthy part of a balanced diet. Unfortunately, not only do we Westerners eat far too much sugar, we consume it, like wheat and dairy, in completely unnatural, highly processed forms. White sugar, brown sugar (which is usually just colored white sugar) and even what is commonly marketed as raw sugar are all refined or processed in some way. While we might not think of sugar as being intelligent as we would a fruit or vegetable, our body cells recognize its structure and can thus process it appropriately. When we consume sugar in foreign forms that depart from their natural state, such as white sugar, it is far more likely to create serious disturbances to the intelligent functioning of our body cells. Over time, the likelihood of cellular ill health must increase. Changing from eating fake white sugar to real whole sugar is one of the simplest ways of improving one's health.

6. Artificial sweeteners

After decades of generally unhealthy diets and lifestyles, of which excessive sugar was just a part, sugar became seen as Public Enemy No.1. Food manufacturers began salivating at this development and thought they would save us from this great evil. They hired food technologists to 'design' healthier alternatives. Although Mother Nature has been feeding the world for millennia, we apparently need food technologists! Quicker than you could become diabetic from drinking commercial softdrinks, a new breed of healthy sugar alternatives was born. Welcome to the world of artificial sweeteners.

As the name implies, artificial sweeteners are exactly that, artificial. Just the name indicates that they are far removed from Mother Nature's health-promoting intelligence. Artificial sweeteners are created in laboratories for the fundamental purpose of stripping off the calories found in real sugar. Basically, the whole business is tied to waistlines and the prospect of losing weight. Artificial sweeteners allow companies to advertise their products as having 'no sugar' (think Coke Zero) and thus have you believe that they are in some way healthy. They are not.

Two of the most prevalent artificial sweeteners are Aspartame, commonly marketed as Nutrasweet or Equal, and Sucralose, commonly marketed as Splenda. Aspartame is found in products like Extra chewing gum, Coke Zero, Diet Coke and Diet Pepsi. Sucralose is present in items such as breakfast bars and softdrinks. Both are included in literally thousands of everyday 'manufactured' foods—as opposed to *real* foods. Though sucralose is made from sugar and aspartame is made from naturally occurring chemicals, their final chemical structures are substantially different from sugar or any foodstuff found in nature. From the understanding of food's vibrational resonance, artificial sweeteners are composed of completely unnatural vibrational energies that are totally foreign to our body's cells. As such, it makes sense that our cells' natural, healthy vibration would likely be greatly disturbed by the regular consumption of such chemicals. It's a bit like introducing the vibration of rap music into a concert of classical music (nothing against rap music of course—yoh!). Importantly, artificial sweeteners are only found in junk foods and have never been a part of the diet of any of the world's healthiest and metabolize people.

What does modern science say about artificial sweeteners? That of course depends on who you listen to. Various medical and government authorities say that artificial sweeteners are perfectly safe. The small print says, 'if consumed in low quantities'. One would assume that this means they can be harmful at high levels! Of course, similar authorities have reassured us in the past that our health was not at risk from suspected chemicals in our agriculture (e.g. DDT), heavy metals in our fish (e.g. mercury) or additives in many of our foods (e.g. sodium nitrite). At the very least, one would want to be cautious. Other researchers and medical experts tell us that aspartame is made from methanol, a highly toxic alcohol, as well as aspartic acid and phenylalanine, two chemicals often considered neurotoxins in high doses. They cite anecdotal and research evidence linking aspartame, for example, to conditions such as headaches, migraines, blurred vision, muscle aches, nausea, memory loss and dizziness right through to cancers and multiple sclerosis.

As with many controversial issues, the science on artificial sweeteners is divided. It really depends on which vested interest you want to listen to. In such instances, rather than getting caught up in the supposed science from either point of view, it can be wise to consult a higher wisdom. The highest wisdom and authority of all as declared by the ancient masters is that of our own inner wisdom. This is discussed in detail in Wisdom Seven, but is pertinent whenever there is some speculation or debate on a matter. Instead of listening to any supposed authority, why not simply ask yourself, 'Does this makes sense? Does this feel right? Is this natural?' In the case of artificial sweeteners, do you believe that chemically altered, artificially manufactured substances (made for profit) are better for your health than small amounts of Mother Nature's unadulterated sugar cane—or other naturally occurring sweeteners?

Interestingly, even apart from the safety issue, there is much debate about whether artificial sweeteners are even effective for weight control. Although they have no calories, those who regularly consume artificial sweeteners often find themselves craving more sweet foods. This is possibly due to the fact that like all processed foods, artificial sweeteners lack the vibrational resonance needed to truly satisfy us on an emotional or a cellular level. In Ayurveda, the purpose of food is to nourish the emotions as well as the body. In many cases, those who rely on artificial sweeteners end up eating more than they otherwise would and thus putting on more weight, because they haven't truly satisfied their desire for the sweet taste in a natural way.

Once again, age-old natural wisdom shouts at us from afar—there is a lot more to health than reducing calories. Artificial sweeteners have nothing to do with natural health. As I repeat consistently, as soon as we start looking at weight loss in isolation from living in tune with the eternal, natural laws of health, we are doomed. If you are going to have something sweet, keep it natural.

From the perspective of whole food nutrition, we can now see that even what we consider healthy these days is often a very poor cousin. A typical salad sandwich bought from the local cafeteria is understandably considered a pretty healthy meal. Let's have a look.

White bread—arghh! Margarine—arghh! 'Processed' meat—arghh! 'Processed' mayonnaise—arghh! Some (hopefully washed) lettuce and tomato that may or may not have been chemically sprayed—that's the healthy part! And finally a sprinkle of common, highly refined table salt that has most of its natural minerals processed out and a few preservatives and artificial anti-caking agents added in—arghh!

Overall, this is probably better than a hamburger and fries, but certainly not ideal. Now before you get too depressed, let's look at some ways to improve things.

Eating more natural whole foods—Ideas to help

Where possible look to buy and consume the following:

1. Whole fruits and vegetables rather than those in plastic, packets or pills
2. Unhomogenized rather than homogenized milks (raw milk is the best of all if you can get it)
3. Whole wheat products—breads, flours, pastas—rather than refined wheat products, like white breads and white flours
4. Wholegrains generally rather than refined grains
5. Organic butter (small amounts), avocado, nut butters or olive oil rather than margarine products
6. Unrefined sea or rock salt rather than regular table salt, e.g. Celtic sea salt or Himalayan crystal rock salt
7. Honey or unrefined sugar rather than white sugar, brown sugar or artificial sweeteners
8. Organic rather than processed meats where meat is eaten. Processed meats have been strongly linked to increased incidence of diseases such as cancer.
9. Non-genetically engineered (GE) foods—GE foods are the absolute antithesis of intelligent foods.

Notes:
- In our modern-day 'wisdom', refined wheat does not even have to be labelled as refined. It just gets labelled as wheat. To get whole wheat, a food company has to label it as such. Weird, isn't it? Look for products that are labelled as whole wheat or wholegrain, not just wheat. Wholegrain is preferable to wholemeal where possible.

- Look for unrefined sugar such as Jaggery, Rapadura, Sucanat or Muscovado (Asian or health food shops best). Instead of drinking skim or low fat milk, boil one part real milk with one part water.

- Avoid foods—if you can call them foods—with the words 'hydrogenated' or 'partially hydrogenated' in the ingredients list

- If you regularly get headaches, migraines, dizziness, muscle aches or other symptoms that you just can't explain, try reducing your consumption of products containing artificial sweeteners and see if your symptoms reduce. Particularly avoid products with aspartame, sucralose and high fructose corn syrup. Look for Sweetener [951] (food labelling code for aspartame) and Sweetener [955] (food labelling code for sucralose). For a complete list, Google 'list of artificial sweeteners'.

- An example of a healthier salad sandwich would be: wholemeal or wholegrain bread, avocado spread and salad of choice that preferably doesn't look like it came out of a tin. If eating meat, fresh meat pieces rather than highly processed sliced meat. A falafel, lentil patty or tofu-type filling may be preferred. No or minimal salt unless you carry your own. (I keep some unrefined rock salt in my car glove box). Can be complemented with a curry, soup or dhal-type dish.

INTELLIGENT FOOD KEY 2—LIFE-FORCE

Though everything at its fundamental level, or close to it, is nothing other than vibrations of energy, the vibrational energy, or frequency of living things, is quite different from that of non-living things. As such, in addition to consuming foods in their whole food form, what time-tested natural health sciences have always considered more important than whether a food contains nutrient A or nutrient B is whether a food is 'alive'. As food in its purest sense is that which gives life, the highest priority as understood by the ancients was whether food had *'life-force'*.

In Ayurveda, the vital life-force that enlivens the air we breathe, the water we drink and the food we eat is known as *'prana'*. While the term prana is often used in reference to the individual breath, in this context it relates to the most basic energy, or primal force, of the universe. Other cultures also have this dual understanding of the life-force, though they know it by different names. The Greeks refer to it as 'pneuma', the Chinese as 'chi' and the Japanese as 'ki'. While most discussion of lifeforce comes about when discussing traditional breathing practices such as pranayama, ancient Eastern cultures understood that the fundamental purpose of eating and drinking was also to imbibe life-force. It is not simply carbohydrates or vitamins that give us life but the more subtle quality of a food's life-force that really enlivens and energizes us.

Old food, leftover food, tinned food or other highly processed foods not only lose their vitamin content, but are usually devoid of life-force. Packaged tomato paste, canned peaches or a reheated risotto from three days ago may all contain some nutrition from a modern scientific perspective, but they are all predominantly 'dead' foods. If we could see their molecular vibration, tomato paste or a week-old spaghetti napolitano would have little or no vibration. In contrast, a fully ripe tomato or a freshly cooked pasta dish would be literally dancing with energy and vitality.

Furthermore, the fact that old or processed foods don't taste like fresh, whole foods creates further problems. In the traditional Eastern medicines, the unique taste of a food is considered fundamental to health and is in itself known to have medicinal effects. Different tastes and textures are required to create balance in our physiologies. When we distort the natural taste and texture of Mother Nature's foods, we begin disrupting our body's natural appetite regulation, satisfaction levels and ability to self-heal. Whole foods that have most of their life-force retained truly nourish our cells at their deepest level. When we eat processed, old, leftover or lifeless foods, our cells literally don't get fed the electro-chemical life energy needed to perform their jobs properly. Thus we are far more likely to feel unsatisfied, to binge eat and/or overeat.

Food by definition is photo-electric energy. Old or processed foods, however, are electrically dead.

If you eat such foods regularly over time, you will get some sub-optimal nutrition, however your cells will not sing. You will feel heavy and dull rather than light and energized.

You won't feel alive because there is no life in your food.

Lifeless foods create 'less life.'

Fresh is best

One of the greatest differences between our diets and those of long-living, traditional cultures is the time difference between when the food is taken from the ground and when it is eaten. Having food fresh is obviously the best way to ensure the highest levels of life-force in our food. Fresh foods are alive.

Just as the cycles of the sun and moon underpin the growth of foods before they are picked, traditional cultures also understood that it is these cycles that govern how quickly the prana, or life-force, in our food is lost. While we think of the sun as giving life and energy, the cycle of the moon (the restful lunar phase) is associated with the opposite qualities. Certain Native American tribes viewed nighttime as the death of the day. This was not just symbolic but true in terms of the subtle cosmic energy that flows through all of life. With the exception of some grains, the quality of a food's life-force was understood to diminish with each cycle of the sun and moon, i.e. each night. Food picked when ripe and eaten on the same day was known to have maximum life-force.

Common practice today has fruits and vegetables being picked weeks before they are even ripe. This not only means sub-optimal life-force, nutrition and flavor, but some vegetables can even be harmful at this time. Mother Nature's cycles of time are not haphazard or governed by chance. They are perfectly designed to ensure the best possible chance of health and survival for all her creatures. As a means of defense, certain fruits and vegetables produce toxins to combat potential threats, such as insects, until they are ready for eating. Though perfectly healthy once ripe, green tomatoes, eggplants, peppers and alfalfa sprouts can contain toxins before they are fully matured. Mother Nature gives us the signs to know when food will be most health-promoting through the smell, taste and feel of the food. The toxins in green tomatoes give them an unpleasant bitter taste—a warning not to eat them in this state. Other foods don't smell right or haven't adequately softened—like most fruit in supermarkets and grocery stores today.

This is not to say that eating fruit and vegetables picked before their optimal time will be toxic. The majority artificially ripen in storage or after being bought. However, Mother Nature has created a recipe for food that has been perfected over millennia, and it is based on immutable laws related to time. Avocadoes need a good nine months to fully grow and ripen. Carrots, depending on the variety and growing conditions, take between two and three months. Wise ancient farmers knew that certain foods were best planted at different times within nature's daily, monthly and seasonal cycles to maximize their goodness. Likewise, foods are also best harvested at specific times ... when they are ripe! When we start messing with Mother Nature's clock, we start messing with our health.

Although many supermarkets claim they sell fresh fruit and vegetables, it's been suggested that some items bought in supermarkets can be up to a year old.[10] Having food picked before its time and then trucked or flown thousands of kilometers before being frozen, stored, thawed, sprayed and shined is certainly more convenient, but it is not the basis of ideal nutrition. In fact, such is the sad state of fresh food these days that many experts suggest frozen food has as much if not more nutritional value by the time we get to eat it. While it is a depressing state of aff airs when we have to consider frozen food as being a healthier alternative, for practical purposes, frozen food that has 'not' been cooked is generally better than old, leftover or tinned food. Such food is probably the best alternative when fresh food is not available. Frozen food that has already been cooked, however, will generally have minimal life-force left and is not ideal.

> Our recent departure from fresh, naturally grown food is no doubt why we are seeing such a resurgence in local farmers' markets, home gardens and even cooperative food gardens in highrise apartment blocks.
>
> This is a wonderful trend and one that we should do everything we can to promote. Innately, we all know that fresh is best.

Microwaved food—'convenient'… but not 'conducive' to optimal health

I debated whether to include this section, as for most busy people any suggestion that microwaves are not particularly healthy is likely to go down about as well as telling Russians that vodka isn't exactly ambrosia. However, as this is a book about health rather than convenience, I felt that it should be included. Of course, you can decide how practical it is for you.

Apart from eating old or highly processed foods, there are two other ways we commonly deplete the life-force in our food. Overcooking it and microwaving it. Overcooking food is a well-established means of reducing its nutrient levels. It is also known to sap its life-force. More serious, however, is the deleterious effect of microwaving food.

It would make sense that if we want to maximize our health and wellbeing naturally, we would want to cook our food in a natural way. According to time-tested sciences such as Ayurveda, for food to be transformed into something that truly nourishes the tissues of our body, it requires the element of 'fire' or fire-related heat. Ayurveda refers to our internal fire, or 'agni', when describing how our bodies digest food. If we eat food that hasn't been cooked, it is our digestive fire which needs to break that food down into its basic constituents in order to make it useful to the body. The ancient Romans saw our body temple as '*a house of fire*' as it is the element of fire which is necessary to transform one substance into another. Fire transforms wood into energy, water into steam, butter into ghee. Cooking food slowly via the element of fire transforms it in a way that promotes its digestion and absorption once inside the body. It also makes the food more palatable and maintains its normal texture without disturbing its nutrition, life-force or inner intelligence. The food retains its natural vibration and thus resonates most harmoniously with the body's inner tissues, promoting health.

Microwaves work by microwave radiation. While we often get scared by the term radiation, radiation is not inherently bad. The sun too works via microwave radiation, however the microwave energy from the sun is distinctly different from microwaves emitted by microwave ovens. Unlike microwaves from the sun, microwave ovens produce what is called '*frictional heat*'. This basically causes the food particles, particularly the water molecules, to resonate at very high frequencies. As such, the food is heated (often unevenly) but it is not truly 'cooked'. At best, the chemical structure of the food is not changed properly, reducing our body's ability to utilize the food's nutritional value. At worst, the excessive friction and high-speed movement of molecules generated by microwaving, which is totally unnatural and not found in any conventional cooking method, can cause surrounding molecules to be severely damaged and thus deformed.

From the perspective of food intelligence, microwaving not only interferes with, but disturbs the intrinsic intelligence of food. As discussed, it is the unique vibrational frequency, or wavelength, of different foods that resonates with and thus strengthens the different cells, tissues and organs of our body. A micro 'wave' is also a wavelength of energy, however it is not one that naturally resonates with the internal orchestra of our body's cells. Furthermore, what microwaves do to the natural taste and texture of our foods would suggest that they are far less than ideal—unless you like uniformly mushy, tasteless food that is half cold and half hot. Again, it is the unique smell, taste and texture of foods that delivers their medicinal effects. As Hippocrates declared, 'food is medicine'. In this light, common sense tells us that a flaccid, flavorless, microwaved carrot cannot compare in nourishing or healing power to a crisp, raw carrot or a naturally cooked one.

What does science say? As usual it's highly divided. There are a number of highly unfavorable research studies, and there are also many industry experts and highly respected bodies such as the CSIRO which say microwaves are perfectly safe. While some research studies suggest that we don't lose out in terms of vitamin and mineral nutrition from microwaving food (many others do), it's good to once again remind ourselves that nutrition involves far more than gross-level nutrients. Also, it is not just how many nutrients a food has according to laboratory analysis that matters, it's how effective those nutrients are in nourishing the cells once they are inside our body. If the natural structure of food molecules becomes distorted, it is not hard to see how regular consumption of such foods can lead not only to compromised nutrition but also to potentially serious problems.

Again, it can be good to simply put the science to one side for a moment and consult our gut wisdom. Does 'zapping' our food in a microwave really constitutes the healthiest way to heat—it's not really cooking—the raw materials that build our entire body? Personally, the fact that we use the terms 'zap' and 'nuke' in reference to microwaves sends a chill up my spine, and suggests to me that something is not as natural, nor possibly as safe as we are told. I suspect that in a future time of higher wisdom, we will find that microwaves cause significantly reduced nutrition, in the true sense of providing life-force, as well as distorting the natural intelligence of our food. Microwaves are unquestionably convenient, and using them every now and then would be unlikely to cause any significant problems. However, it is hard to see their regular use as anything but a significant compromise to one's long-term health.

Maybe the most enlightened recommendation on the matter goes to Cyndi O'Meara, one of Australia's most well-known and respected nutritionists. Cyndi says, 'If you have a microwave at all, put it out in your garage to heat your heat packs.'

Maximizing life-force—Ideas to help

If you are reading this and largely live on leftovers, supermarket fare, microwaved or frozen food, don't stress. Eating wholesome, fresh foods in our modern world is certainly a challenge, to say the least. However, look to implement one or two of the following changes to gradually increase the life-force in your food.

1. Consider growing some of your own vegetables at home. Little vegie patches are not as hard work as you might expect. Once set up, they can save you considerable money, are infinitely healthier, and are a great way to reconnect to nature.
2. If you can't grow your own vegies, look at teaming up with neighbors or friends who grow theirs and start a communal natural food cooperative. Food is a great way to help reconnect communities.
3. If neither of the above ideas is practical, where possible buy your fruit and vegetables from a local growers' market. Often there are lists of local farmers' markets in health food shops or on local natural health websites.
4. Otherwise, purchase from your local green grocer, but find out what day they receive their delivery and try to buy on that day. This will ensure you get the freshest produce possible.
5. Consume anything in cans, tins or plastic sparingly. Get some recipe books on how to make simple, quick meals out of basic, natural produce—anything Jamie Oliver does is usually good, as he is all about getting back to eating simple, real foods.
6. Avoid or reduce leftovers as much as possible, particularly where food is left overnight or frozen and reheated on a subsequent day. Food that is eaten later the same day that it was cooked will lose some life-force but is generally okay.

7. If you regularly eat pre-packaged frozen meals, gradually replace some of these with freshly cooked meals.

8. Minimize or avoid microwaves as much as possible. Favor conventional methods of steaming, boiling, grilling and oven baking. Think of the extra time needed to cook your food naturally as one of the best investments in your health.

9. Buy yourself a juicer and start your day with a life-force boost of fresh vegetable and/or fruit juice.

10. Try to eat high-intelligence, high life-force food as much as possible when you are home so you can just relax and not worry too much when having to consume processed or microwaved food away from home.

INTELLIGENT FOOD KEY 3—VARIETY

Have you ever marvelled at the almost infinite variety of Mother Nature's foods? Our earth, Mother Nature's body, is a veritable smorgasbord. She is an almost endless banquet of different kinds of fruits, vegetables, nuts, seeds, grains and other foodstuffs. Importantly, there is a perfect purpose for all this abundance. Mother Nature has provided such a variety of foods to make it easy for us to get all the essential nutrition we need. When we simply eat a sufficient variety of them in their whole food form, we go a long way to getting everything we need in terms of optimal nutrition.

It is such a simple idea, but one that so many of us fail to put into practice. Most people wouldn't even be able to remember the last time they ate some sesame, sunflower or pumpkin seeds. Legumes (beans, lentils) are often a greater source of derision and humor than they are a bountiful and nourishing source of nutrition. Most people don't even know that quinoa and burghul are actually foods, let alone know how nutritious they are. Some people might eat salted cashews every now and then, but how many people regularly eat macadamia nuts, brazil nuts, hazelnuts, almonds or walnuts?

The reality is that in our ever-increasing desire for fast, ready-made, instantly gratifying foods, we often lose sight of Mother Nature's vast array of health-promoting foods. Instead of consuming even a reasonable variety of the natural foods on offer, we have been brainwashed into believing that it is impossible to get optimal nutrition from food and that we have to take copious supplements. However, everyday nuts and seeds provide many of the common minerals many people are deficient in. Simply by eating a wider selection of fruits and vegetables—other than the usual apples, bananas, potatoes and carrots—some people could save thousands of dollars on 'super' juices and laboratory manufactured anti-oxidants.

When health authorities suggest we reduce our red meat intake in order to cut our risk of heart disease and cancer, some nutritionists—and especially the meat lobby—tell us we will be subjecting ourselves to almost certain iron and protein deficiencies. If the rest of our diet consists of breakfast cereals, white bread sandwiches, an aversion to legumes and includes only the occasional lifeless green vegetable or two, then this might be the case. However, nuts are great for protein and healthy fats. Seeds are loaded with vitamins and trace minerals. Beans and lentils are excellent protein sources. Leafy greens are high in iron and folate. Grains such as barley, oats, quinoa, buckwheat and rye provide excellent all-round nutrition.

> The reality is that if we simply ate more whole foods and supplemented them with different types of nuts, seeds, beans and lentils, a few other grains besides rice and wheat and plenty of leafy greens, vitamin, mineral and general nutrient deficiencies would pretty well cease to exist.

Herbs and spices—variety bursting with intelligence

One of the simplest yet most overlooked (forgotten) practices for expanding our nutritional intake, promoting internal balance and protecting ourselves against disease is the use of everyday herbs and spices. While we in the West are only just starting to uncover some of the outstanding medicinal properties of common herbs and spices, ancient records of their profound healing properties date back well over 5000 years. Natural health sciences with comprehensive herbal medicine systems, such as Ayurvedic Medicine, Tibetan Medicine, Traditional Chinese Medicine and Arabic Medicine, have for many centuries had texts detailing the most comprehensive herbal pharmacopeias.

Herbs and spices both come from plants. Herbs come from the leaves of plants without woody stems. Spices generally come from the roots, bark, seeds, flowers or fruits. From the ancients' understanding, herbs and spices were literally seen as 'concentrated packets of intelligence and life-force'. For this reason they were considered 'manna from heaven' and the powerhouses of Mother Nature's medicine cabinet. The reason we need only small quantities of herbs and spices in comparison to fruits and vegetables is that they are so concentrated. They are literally jam-packed with Mother Nature's healing intelligence.

Although many of us today consider herbs and spices merely in the light of adding certain flavors, aromas or aesthetics to food (or in some cases when ordering Kentucky Fried Chicken), indigenous cultures have known that they can help prevent disease, medicinally heal and optimize mental and physical functioning. A recent supplement of 'The Medical Journal of Australia' has begun reporting some of these effects.[11] Even in these early stages of modern science's research into their effects, we know they can mitigate or fight certain types of cancer cells, neutralize free radical damage, reduce blood sugars, break down fats, stimulate memory, enliven brain function, and strengthen the heart, liver and kidneys. When most of us think of the best sources of anti-oxidants, colored fruits and supplements containing vitamin C, vitamin E or beta carotene generally come to mind. However, oregano, cloves, cinnamon, thyme, rosemary and mint have been shown to be more concentrated sources of anti-oxidants than most fruits and vegetables[12,] and the free-radical scavenging effects of everyday turmeric is many times more powerful gram for gram than vitamin A, C or E.[13]

> In terms of their vibrational resonance, herbs and spices are like concentrated, harmonizing energies. They are medicinal powerhouses that re-tune our body cells, organs and tissues back to their optimal health-promoting frequency.

Six common herbs and spices to smarten up your diet

Turmeric

Turmeric is that funny little orangy powder that has been sitting untouched in most people's spice rack since the end of the First World War. However, there is a good reason Indians have been putting it in their curries for thousands of years. Turmeric is a natural antihistamine, antibiotic, anti-inflammatory, anti-ulcerative and antiseptic. It is renowned for purifying the blood and liver, helping the body to process and neutralize toxins and impurities such as fatty food, cigarette smoke and alcohol. As well as being an antioxidant powerhouse, turmeric has been shown to be a powerful anti-cancer spice and to decrease cardiovascular risk.[14] Curcumin, one of the many active constituents in turmeric, has even been shown to reduce the most common expression of the genetic defect thought to be responsible for cystic fibrosis.[15]

For thousands of years, Ayurveda and other ancient medical systems have prescribed turmeric in certain cases for such conditions, as well as for liver damage, skin conditions and diabetes.

Ginger

Ginger is often called *vishwabhesaj* meaning *'the universal medicine'*.

Ginger can be fresh, like the punnets of ginger you might see in your fruit and vegetable store, or dried, as you would buy in a spice bag or bottle. Fresh ginger is great for stimulating appetite and digestion. It has anti-platelet properties (reduces blood clotting) and powerful anti-inflammatory effects. It can work brilliantly in reducing things like nausea, morning sickness, bronchitis and asthma, and is helpful for circulation, protecting against colds and coughs and respiratory conditions. It can also be excellent for reducing gas and bloating and for settling indigestion.

Cinnamon

Cinnamon is a seemingly innocuous herb. However, like turmeric, it is a highly potent antioxidant. It is warming and sweet by nature and is good for digestion, the kidneys, blood flow and general strength. Arguably its most important use in today's world of skyrocketing diabetes relates to its effects on blood sugars. Recent research has demonstrated that intakes of as little as 1g of cinnamon per day can reduce blood sugars by around 20%, and lower LDL cholesterol (often called 'bad' cholesterol) and total cholesterol in people with type 2 diabetes.[16] Cinnamon has also been prescribed for similar purposes for centuries.

Basil (fresh)

Fresh basil is considered one of the most sacred plants on earth. Easily bought at any grocery shop, basil is great for the nervous, digestive and respiratory systems. It is also prized for its effect in enlivening the mind and aiding memory. It is antibacterial and antiseptic and useful for respiratory or nasal congestion-type problems including colds and flu.

Coriander

Coriander (fresh) is another simple yet powerful health-promoting herb readily available at any grocer. It is good for the digestive, respiratory and urinary systems.

Cardamom

Cardamom is a sweet, warming herb that is good for the stomach and lungs as well as settling the mind.

While modern science is now showing the tremendous benefits of individual herbs and spices, what ancient cultures also knew was that they are even more powerful when combined. Using Mother Nature's principle of synergies, when we combine different herbs and spices, the healing and health-promoting benefits can be magnified many times. The active constituents of turmeric can work wonders within the cells and tissues for breaking down excess fats, however, if it is not well absorbed or is blocked from getting to where it needs to, its effect is severely compromised. When combined with a little black pepper, which is known to stimulate metabolism and help open up the subtle channels of the body, the effects of turmeric can be magnified many times. Similar benefits work for many other herb and spice combinations. Fortunately, we don't need to intellectually understand or wait for modern science to prove the synergistic effects that traditional cultures have known for thousands of years. Simply by combining various herbs and spices that are pleasing to your sense of smell and taste, i.e. you enjoy them, you will naturally receive a number of synergistic benefits.

The real beauty with herbs and spices is that they don't just provide wonderful flavors and nutritional benefits. They can stimulate our appetite, strengthen our digestion, open up the body's subtle channels, and assist with all stages of converting food into healthy tissues and high energy.

Increasing food variety—Ideas to help

1. Buy some seeds, e.g. sunflower, pumpkin, sesame, linseed/flaxseed and add them to various dishes. Sunflower and pumpkin seeds can be dry roasted for one to two minutes and eaten with a sprinkle of salt as a great appetizer. Flaxseeds and sesame can be sprinkled on top of many foods. Flaxseeds are best ground up fresh every few days. Small electric grinders make this easy.

2. Put some nuts in a little tupperware container and carry them in your bag or car to eat instead of junk food if you get hungry between meals.

3. Buy different varieties of nuts—brazil nuts, pistachios, walnuts, macadamias, almonds, hazelnuts. You can also buy ground nuts—or grind your own—and sprinkle them on meals.

4. If you currently screw your face up at the thought of eating legumes, try adding a legume dish or side dish to a meal every now and then. Get yourself a recipe book and try some type of beans, e.g. kidney beans, lima beans, mung beans or *lentils*, e.g. red lentils, brown lentils, green lentils. Nachos or burgers made with lentils or beans can be a good place to start, especially if cooking for kids.

5. Introduce a different type of grain every now and then. This could be a barley soup, biscuits with rolled oats, semolina porridge, or the occasional buckwheat or rye bread.

6. Add more everyday herbs and spices into your diet.

What's possible with an intelligent food diet—the long-living Okinawans

Ishoku-dogan

an Okinawan saying that means *'Food and medicine have the same source.'*

The Southern Japanese prefecture of Okinawa is home to the world's most thoroughly researched long-living population. Until recently, elderly Okinawans enjoyed not only what was the world's longest life expectancy but also the world's longest health expectancy.[17] Unlike the long-living Hunzans, Vilcabambans and Abkhasians, whose ages are often overinflated, the accuracy of the Okinawans' longevity is unquestionable as their ages are validated through the *koseki*, the Japanese family registration system.

Despite becoming highly industrialized, and thus missing out on many of the pristine, unpolluted environmental conditions most other long-living cultures enjoy, the Okinawans have been renowned for their longevity. They have had up to five times the number of centenarians found in most developed countries.[18] More importantly, elderly Okinawans have commonly remained healthy, strong and vital beyond 100 years of age. Even at such ages they have continued to farm, be active and play with their great-great-grandchildren—often up until the last year or so of their lives.

The authors of the world famous Okinawa Centenarian Study showed the Okinawans had among the lowest mortality rates in the world. Coronary heart disease risk was up to 80% less than in the United States. They also had 80% less prostate and breast cancer, more than 50% less colon and ovarian cancer, 40% fewer hip fractures as well as a lower incidence of strokes, dementia, menopausal difficulties and a range of other age-related problems.[19] In one case, an autopsy on a female centenarian showed that her coronary arteries were 'virtually free of atherosclerotic plaque.'[20]

While common factors such as heredity, regular exercise, strong social and family bonds and relatively stress-free living are given for the remarkable aging of the Okinawans, one of the most distinguishing reasons cited is their exceptionally simple and healthful diet. So successful is this way of eating, a book based on its principles, 'The Okinawa Diet Plan', has become a best seller.[21] Traditionally, in addition to consuming a low number of total calories generally, the Okinawan diet was based on:

- minimal or no processed foods (i.e. predominantly 'whole foods')
- almost entirely fresh, seasonal and locally grown produce (high 'life-force')
- a high proportion of their diet as healthy complex carbohydrates—whole grains, fruits and vegetables
- various nuts and seeds
- regular small intakes of fresh fish, but minimal meat or eggs
- a good 'variety' of foods generally[22]

It seems no coincidence that the people who enjoyed one of the longest properly verified life expectancies also consumed one of the most naturally intelligent diets. Unfortunately, things are changing. In a 2003 review of the longevity and diet in Okinawa, as reported in the Asia Pacific Journal of Public Health, the authors note that Okinawans now have life expectancies no higher than the national average for Japan. In their discussion of possible reasons for this change, they note that between 1988 and 1998, the daily intake of meat had increased while the daily intake of pulses and green and yellow vegetables—which were originally about 30% and 50% higher than the national average respectively—had declined to the level of the national average.[23]

With the ever-growing modernization of Okinawa, younger Okinawans are quickly forsaking the traditional diet of their elders in favor of more fast, processed foods. Researchers overseeing this shift are seeing a direct correlation between the amount of Western foods being eaten and the rapid rise in disease now commonly being experienced by younger Okinawans. Photographs of slim, vibrant 100-year-old elders sitting next to obese teenagers paint a very sad picture of the rapid decline in Okinawan health as they move away from eating natural foods. They also provide a poignant reminder to us about what foods should make up the bulk of our shopping carts if we want to promote our highest level of health.

Common food confusions simplified

In light of the understanding of food intelligence, we can now put into perspective some of the food issues that commonly cause confusion in today's world.

The organic versus non-organic food debate

So how does organic food fit in with food intelligence? Organic food simply means that the food is grown without such things as artificial pesticides, fertilisers, hormones or antibiotics.

While this is certainly a good thing, it is important not to automatically equate organic food with high-intelligence food. While most people think of organic food as the healthiest option, you can still buy organic foods that are either highly processed or not fresh. Many breakfast cereals which now market themselves as being organic are still highly processed, old, dead, unhealthy foods. Just because some of the ingredients were grown organically, it doesn't mean that they have any semblance of life-force, or intelligence, once you buy them. Just because the fruit and vegetables you buy are organic, it won't matter much if they are three weeks old by the time you eat them.

This is not to suggest buying organic is not to be recommended. Having food that is grown in soils that have more of their natural fertility still intact, does not require your body to deal with loads of unwanted chemicals, and is more likely to be picked when ripe (rather than weeks early), is certainly a good thing. However, don't focus on going organic at the expense of eating food that isn't fresh or is highly processed. Fresh, non-organic whole foods are far better than organic foods that are highly processed or have lost their life-force.

> **Keep the following grading system in mind when buying food.**
>
> - A grade—fresh, organic, unprocessed (or minimally processed)
> - B grade—fresh, non-organic, minimally processed
> - C grade—organic, minimally processed but not fully fresh
> - D grade—non-fresh, non-organic, processed

Low GI diets

The current fad of glycemic index (GI) foods is an example of the excessive confusion, complexity and time-wasting we create for ourselves when we eat predominantly unnatural, processed foods instead of natural, whole foods. GI is an indicator of the rate at which different foods increase blood sugar levels. Eating high GI foods means our blood sugar levels will tend to rise quickly whereas low GI foods take longer to break down, resulting in lower, more stable sugar levels. Eating a higher percentage of low GI foods is recommended, particularly for diabetics or those with borderline blood sugar levels.

The theory of low GI diets is absolutely fine, but the subsequent need to analyze and assess every food item, based on one isolated effect on our body, is remarkably complicated, hard work, basically unnecessary and sometimes even misleading.

Traditional cultures with the highest percentages of long-living people, who have had little or no incidence of diseases such as obesity or diabetes, have also had absolutely no concept of GI foods. They have simply eaten whole, unrefined foods direct from Mother Nature's kitchen. Most whole foods are predominantly low GI foods. Those that are not, when eaten as part of a 'varied', balanced diet, combine to produce an overall healthy GI and blood sugar level.

At a doctors' conference in 2009, I gave a talk on wellbeing, including the importance of eating natural foods. A doctor came up to me after the presentation to talk to me about GI foods. He was lamenting the fact that rice and pasta were not low GI foods and so he couldn't eat them. The fact that he wasn't overweight or diabetic intrigued me, but nevertheless I pointed out that wholegrain rice and traditional long-grain rice varieties such as basmati, have relatively low GI's and have been a staple of healthy individuals' diets throughout the ages. However, my main point was that it is not foods in isolation that is important. Modern science loves to break things down and analyze them individually, but it's the 'combined effect' of foods that matters. Who eats rice, pasta or bread by itself? Bread in its whole wheat form drizzled with extra virgin olive oil and spread with avocado is by no means a high GI snack. Wholemeal pasta, cooked 'al dente' with lots of vegetables (most of which are low GI), is also a perfectly healthy meal for most people. In many countries, long-grain rice has been eaten with lentils (dhal) and vegetables for centuries. The overall result, which is what's important, is a high intelligence meal, low in GI with a good mix of carbohydrate and proteins.

All other factors being equal, eating even a reasonable variety of natural whole foods and ditching junk, processed foods will ensure optimal blood sugars without any need to analyze every morsel of food put in your mouth.

This is not to criticize the vast number of low GI cookbooks or experts who promote them, it's just that Mother Nature never designed healthy eating to be that complicated.

Low carb diets

Low carbohydrate (low carb) diets are another modern-day fad that has been all the rage in recent times. They have been promoted based on the assumption that carbohydrates are bad for our waistlines and weight. Unfortunately, the whole argument for low carb diets again misses the essential wisdom of food and nutrition. The problem is not the consumption of carbohydrates. The problem stems from most people consuming carbohydrates in their highly refined, unintelligent forms. Unlike refined carbohydrates, carbohydrates eaten in their natural, unprocessed forms—even supposedly bad, starchy carbs such as bread, rice and pasta—do not cause the same irregular spikes in blood sugar and insulin production. As such, they tend to be directed to important biological processes such as energy production and temperature regulation, and not simply stored as extra body fat as refined carbohydrates tend to be.

Rather than detailing the folly and even the potential dangers of low carb diets here (a full discussion is included in the ebook), the following observation should help put things into perspective.

The two biggest populations of slim people on the earth in recent times—the Chinese and Indians—and every one of the long-living, low-disease cultures cited throughout this book, e.g. the Okinawans, Hunzans, Vilcabambans, Abkhasians, Campodimele and Symiots, have all consumed 'high carbohydrate' diets.

They have just eaten them in their natural forms. This means wholegrain rice, wholegrain breads, fruits and vegetables rather than refined pastas, refined rice, refined breads and packaged fruits.

Eating intelligent food in the real world—a practical 80% goal

While the theory of eating intelligent, natural foods makes good sense, for most people it is almost impossible to live in our modern world and eat no processed or slightly old foods. We have to be practical and enjoy life. Being happy and relatively stress-free should always be paramount. Don't beat yourself up if you can't eat a completely 'intelligent' food diet. In fact, it can be perfectly healthy to let your hair down a bit every now and then. The 'occasional' fast food junk-fest, chocolate craving or potato chip indulgence (my personal favorite, just ahead of butterscotch and honeycomb ice-cream in summer) is unlikely to cause any major problems. However, by regularly consuming such 'intelligence depleted' foods, we must greatly increase our chances of experiencing compromised health over time.

Commonsense suggests that there is a balance point between what is necessary for us to maintain good health and still being able to live practically in our modern world. I believe the tipping point towards illness is likely to occur around the point of having more than 20% of our diet as processed or old food. Therefore, where possible, work towards achieving 'the 80% goal' as outlined below.

1. Have at least 80% of your diet as whole foods.

Consume less food in processed forms, e.g. packaged foods, cookies, crackers, refined sugars or white flour.

2. Have at least 80% of your diet as plant foods.

Meat can be considered an old or life-force diminished food as it comes from 'dead' animals. The large majority of the world's metabolize cultures have eaten meat in small amounts, if at all—usually as a side dish or as part of special celebrations. Those that have had high meat intakes generally consumed it from wild, naturally fed animals and had far higher daily activity levels than we do today. Physical activity enhances the body's ability to process heavier, harder-to-digest meats and to eliminate their toxic residues before they create problems in the body. If you eat a lot of meat, begin cutting out processed meats. Then gradually reduce your meat portions and increase your servings of legumes, grains, fruits, vegetables, nuts and seeds.

3. Have at least 80% of your diet as fresh foods.

Consume less food that is old or life-force depleted, e.g. leftovers, canned foods or microwaved foods.

* Eating an 80+ percent intelligent-food diet is not always easy. Work towards the highest intelligence diet you can, but not to the point of sabotaging your enjoyment of life.

The following table can be used as a quick reference guide for making more intelligent food choices.

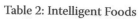

Table 2: Intelligent Foods

Low-intelligence food examples (Avoid / Reduce)	High-intelligence food examples (Favor)
Refined breads/flours—white bread, white flour	Wholegrain or wholemeal breads, atta flour, wholemeal flour, spelt flour
Other refined grains	Wholemeal pasta, basmati or wholegrain rice, rolled oats, wholegrain rye
Processed breakfast cereals—most are full of sugar and devoid of intelligence and life-force	Porridge (rolled oats, semolina, wholegrain rye), homemade or minimally processed muesli, bircher muesli, cooked apples/ pears with spices and dry roasted nuts and seeds
Margarine or margarine spreads* or any foods with trans fats or PVHO's	Olive oil, avocado, nut butters, tahini. Butter or ghee in small quantities
Processed milks—homogenized milks, artificially fortified skim milks	Unhomogenized full cream milk. * Always boil milk and if concerned about weight gain, drink it sparingly and dilute it with water (i.e. half milk, half water) rather than use skim milks
Refined sugars (white sugar, brown sugar) and artificial sweeteners, e.g. aspartame [951], sucralose [955]	Honey, molasses, unprocessed sugar (ask for jaggery, rapadura, muscovado or sucanat)
Sweets (biscuits, cakes) made with artificial ingredients, e.g. egg substitutes, fruit flavorings	Sweets, cakes or biscuits with real ingredients such as raw, unhomogenized milk, real butter, real fruit, real cocoa or real vanilla
Processed salt, e.g. regular table salt	Unprocessed rock or sea salt, crystal salt
Packaged food—food in cans, tins, plastic containers, e.g. pre-cooked meals, tinned baked beans, canned asparagus, frozen peas, fruit bars, fruit in plastic containers	Food as it grows on trees or comes out of the earth. Real bananas, apples, pears, oranges kiwi fruits, carrots, broccoli, tomatoes, spinach, cauliflower, nuts, beans, grains etc

Low-intelligence food examples (Avoid / Reduce)	High-intelligence food examples (Favor)
Old foods, e.g. supermarket produce, old (yellow) cheeses, old processed yoghurts	Fresh foods—where possible, home grown or local market produce eaten soon after picking. Fresh, soft cheeses, fresh yoghurts, etc
Processed meats, e.g. ham, salami, sliced turkey	Organic meat if eaten (small quantities)
Limited variety of foods	Staple foods complemented with a variety of nuts, e.g. almonds, macadamias, brazil, walnuts, hazelnuts seeds, e.g. linseed/flaxseed, sesame, pumpkin, sunflower legumes, e.g. various beans, lentils/dhals
Chutneys, sauces, jams with sugar as the first ingredient	Chutneys, sauces, jams with the main ingredient listed first, e.g. strawberries in strawberry jam, mangoes in mango chutney
Chocolate—commercial chocolates that are full of chemicals and milk solids	Organic chocolate if eaten (e.g. Green & Blacks) or higher quality European chocolate
Bottled herbs and minimal use of spices	Fresh herbs, e.g. parsley, basil, coriander. Regular use of spices, e.g. ginger, turmeric, cumin, cardamom, cinnamon
Chemically laden food	Organic food if practical (though having food fresh and unprocessed is more important than it being organic)
Microwaved food	Conventionally/naturally cooked, e.g. steamed, boiled, oven-baked
Genetically modified foods (GMO Foods)	Non-GMO foods—avoid GMO foods like the plague
Nano foods—any food based on nanotechnology (this is completely unnatural)	Natural, non-manipulated foods

Seed wisdom

As I write this, there are dozens of traditional cultures throughout the world who have lived relatively long, healthy lives, with few of the health problems we commonly experience in the West. How much do they know about GI foods, good and bad fats, or what foods are high in anti-oxidants, polyphenols and bioflavonoids? Nothing, they have never even heard of them. Similarly, animals have absolutely no concept of calories, good or bad carbohydrates or low fat foods. Many years ago a group of animals was observed in the wild. They were given access to an abundant food supply and were simply observed without any human intervention. They could eat whatever they wanted, whenever they wanted and in whatever quantity they desired.

What percentage of the animals do you think became obese?
0%.

What percentage developed a nutritional deficiency?
0%.

What percentage became diabetic?
0%

What percentage became depressed?
Well, this wasn't actually assessed, but I'd be guessing it to be 0% ... except maybe for the wombats—they always look a bit depressed!

I believe that the essence of observations such as these is that we simply need to get back a little closer to Mother Nature. Food, nutrition and healthy eating are really much simpler than we have made it. So-called foods such as white flour, artificial sweeteners, homogenized milk, refined sweets and genetically engineered foods are not real foods. They are *fake foods*. We call them food, but they do not do what food is designed to do—to truly enliven our body's inner intelligence and strengthen the natural, harmonious vibration of our cellular orchestra. While we can't always escape these foods, if we want our bodies to work intelligently, we predominantly need to eat intelligent foods—natural foods that have nourished the human race since the dawn of time.

Every now and then, stop, sit down, relax and take a deep breath. Bite into a fresh organic carrot or a perfectly ripe mango and really taste it. Chew it fully and let the essence of it register with your inner orchestra. Take the time to rekindle your connection to Mother Nature's foods. Begin to take pleasure in them. Find joy in them beyond their gross level taste. Delight in the infinite variety of natural foods and experiment with the different blends, textures and flavors.

> Fall in love with Mother Nature's intelligent foods and your body will begin to resonate like a beautiful orchestra—a musical masterpiece far more rapturous than any of Mozart's or Beethoven's greatest works.

* More information on eating intelligent foods has been included for you in the ebook. See markbunn.com.au/awmh1_ebook. This includes simple ways to get more herbs and spices into your diet, a comprehensive discussion of low carb diets, and an additional copy of the 'Table of Intelligent Foods' that can be printed off and kept in your kitchen for easy reference.

Wisdom Four

Exercise in Ways that Unite Mind, Body and Spirit

Walking to work can be an unavoidable waste of time. It can also be an adventure in movement and balance. Cleaning the kitchen can be a chore. It can also be an intricate dance. Numbed to everything except results, we are likely to miss the dance. But what are results? We get to work. The walk between home and work was a meaningless interval. The kitchen is clean. It will be dirty again tomorrow. We have built the tallest building, the longest expressway, the biggest cities. We have won the game. But how did we feel from inside while we were doing it? Did we dance?
George Leonard in 'The Ultimate Athlete"

n August 1993, a group of middle-aged Native American Indians was invited to run in a 100-mile race through the Colorado Mountains (Leadville) alongside a number of world-class athletes. Why on earth would the organizers of the race do such a thing? Was it some sort of joke? Was it some sort of strange cross-cultural gesture—or were they simply trying to embarrass or even kill them?

They did it because word had spread to North America that there was a tribe of Native Americans that had gained a God-like reputation for their remarkable, almost supernatural feats of endurance. There had been stories of individuals running for days on end, covering hundreds of miles to deliver messages to a neighboring tribe, only to stop for a short time, turn around and run right back. American athletic authorities were understandably intrigued, if not skeptical, to say the least. To run such distances in extremely mountainous terrain and under challenging conditions was almost incomprehensible. How could such 'simple' people, without any modern training or the latest scientific technologies, possibly achieve such feats? So the authorities thought they would test these supposedly superhuman runners themselves and invited—or rather challenged—them to participate in some of their races.

In the early hours of a fresh Colorado morning, five Native American Indians wearing bright, colorful traditional dress set off at the back of a field of some 300 elite runners.[2] Rejecting the Americans' offers of the latest high-tech running shoes, they wore sandals made out of old tyres. Their fuel was not Gatorade or some high energy sports drink but homemade pinole—roasted corn ground and mixed with water. While the elite athletes went out hard and led early, the Native Americans seemed not to be in any great rush. They shuffled along from the start, almost in cruise control and seemingly oblivious to the fact that this was supposed to be a race.

As the hours passed, however, the leading athletes began to wane. Their enthusiastic start gradually slowed to a somewhat tired pace. The Indians shuffl ed along at the same speed, seemingly without effort and certainly showing no signs of pain, discomfort or fatigue. A few hours on, much to everyone's surprise, the Native American elders seemed to be gaining ground. After a few more hours, they began overtaking their younger, more highly trained fellow competitors. The longer the race went, the greater the contrast between the exhausted, conventional athletes, who were pushing themselves to the limit, and their traditional counterparts, who looked more and more as if they were on a leisurely Sunday afternoon stroll.

First across the line in a time of 20 hours and 20 minutes was ... '55 *year-old*" Native American Victoriano. Not bad! 30 minutes later in second place was Ceraldo, another Native American. Both runners set new race records.[3] Most interesting was that the victors did not show any outward signs of distress. In fact, whereas the other competitors finished the race sprawling across the line and crashing in an exhausted heap, Victoriano and Ceraldo looked as if they could just as easily do the whole thing again. Scientists have since measured the heart rates and blood pressures of such runners after similar races and found them to have returned to pre-race levels (or lower) within minutes of finishing.

How could this be and what does it have to do with healthy exercise? To understand it and learn some valuable lessons for our own health and experience with exercise, it is good to appreciate the background of these impressive runners. They know themselves as *Raramuri*, though most people know them as the *Tarahumara Indians*. This is what the Spanish originally called them when they settled nearby. 'Tarahumara' literally means *'foot runners'*. 'Raramuri' also equates to 'runners' in their own native language. Living for thousands of years in the Sierra Madre mountains, a few hundred kilometers south of the US border in northwest Mexico, and more recently in the more remote Copper Canyon region, their whole existence has been founded on the ability to travel vast distances on foot. Children as young as three or four years of age can walk five or six kilometers at a time. As they grow up, running becomes an integral and special part of life. For the Tarahumara, running is entwined into their religious ceremonies and is their sole means of communicating with neighboring tribes, most of which are many kilometers away. Along with dancing, the activities of walking and running are associated with the enjoyment and fun of intertribal interaction.

The point of all this is not that we should try to emulate these people just because they show remarkable feats of endurance. We simply do not need to do this. Our lifestyles, fortunately in many ways, are not conducive to developing such feats of physical prowess. However, it does highlight the possibility that our modern way of exercising might not be ideal.

> In contrast to the short-term 'stress and strain' approach of much of our conventional exercise practices, the Tarahumara serve as a modern-day reminder of many ancient traditions which saw exercise as a means to cultivating higher states of awareness rather than simply bigger biceps or a firmer backside.
>
> They also remind us of the more enlightening benefits of exercise when performed for enjoyment and pleasure rather than purely for weight loss, an adrenaline rush, or just because we are 'supposed to'.

Ancient view of exercise—for mind and spirit not just the body

From the earliest recorded histories, physical activity has played a prominent role in the peak development of humankind. However, in most of the more developed and wisest of the ancient cultures, the importance of exercise went far beyond mere physical benefits. The traditional view of human life was as an amalgamation of mind, body and soul. Exercise was largely seen as a way of fostering and promoting the interrelationship and harmony between these three aspects of one's life.

From the ancient Greek viewpoint, the human body was a *'temple housing the mind and soul'*. Practices such as gymnastics, which were a large part of the earliest Olympics, were performed to maximize the physical and mental aspects of the body temple. Though we usually think of philosophy as a somewhat cerebral activity, many famous ancient philosophers including Pythagoras, Plato and Aristotle were diligent exercise enthusiasts. They knew that a fit and healthy body was integral to cultivating higher creativity, insight, intuition and even spiritual development. Ancient Egyptians were known to practice special physical postures similar to what we know as yoga. However, their goal was not simply physical flexibility or strength, but also, and more importantly, to develop spiritual awareness and inner enlightenment.

In the West today, martial arts are often associated with fighting, aggression and even violence. However, the ancient practice of martial arts was originally designed as a spiritual exercise. With its Eastern roots dating back well into ancient times, its true purpose was not to defeat, conquer or pulverise some external opponent. Rather it was to conquer one's inner demons and become master of one's own mind and body. In their original form, martial arts were an internal, spiritually based practice, far removed from most of the martial arts we see in the West today. The Shaolin Monks, one of the true embodiments not only of martial arts but also of what we could call enlightened exercise, beautifully explain the underlying philosophy of their training when they declare:

The spiritual controls the physical. One's spirit controls one's body.

He who conquers is strong.
He who conquers himself is mighty.

In addition to going to churches, temples and ashrams to find inner peace and spiritual salvation, the ancients felt that exercise could also provide transcendental experiences. Indeed, done in the right way, they saw it as a gateway to God—as powerful as any spiritual retreat or religious revival meeting.

The ultimate purpose of exercise—getting 'in the ZONE'

In the ancient Vedic philosophy dating back thousands of years, the highest goal in life was to unlock our limitless potential, grow to higher states of consciousness, and ultimately to live in complete harmony with the universal, or cosmic intelligence. As a result, everything one did in life was designed to promote such growth and experiences. Exercise was no different. In fact it was seen as one of the most powerful ways to cultivate our highest state of mind and body integration, and even promote spiritual enlightenment.

This state of peak integration was understood as a coexistence of opposites. It involves being dynamically engaged in activity while simultaneously enjoying an inner silence and calm. The 'zone' experience in exercise is really just a temporary taste of this stress-free style of functioning and provides a glimpse into the higher, mostly untapped states of human consciousness.

Traditionally, the role of physical exercise was often seen as an extension of the inner mental practice of meditation. With deep silence and relaxation within activity as the supreme goal, meditation cultured this state from the level of the mind, while 'proper' exercise cultured it from the level of the body.

When one engages in an appropriate meditation practice, the inner peace and silence developed gets integrated with the more efficient functioning of the body developed from proper exercise. In time, a state of inner calm and stress-free functioning begins to occur simultaneously with outer dynamic activity. What we currently know as the almost mystical zone or exercise-high experience—which is far more than simply an endorphin high—was the central and often sole goal of ancient exercise practices. While we consider these peak states of performance as seemingly inexplicable, once-in-a-lifetime experiences, they were once the very purpose and expected outcome of engaging in exercise.

When we exercise or perform activities that unify rather than stress our mind and body, we naturally create more 'flow state', or exercise-high, experiences. Ironically, in this light, stress and fatigue, the pillars of Western exercise, are seen to be the only things that actually stop us from enjoying the ultimate exercise experience.

The experience of being totally involved in an activity or exercise—*the flow*—was not traditionally seen as a stroke of good fortune or a rare, mystical occurrence. It was seen as the natural by-product of a properly functioning physiology performing appropriate exercise.[a]

Modern-day exercise—the myth of 'No Pain, No Gain'

If it weren't for the fact that the TV set and the refrigerator are so far apart, some of us wouldn't get any exercise at all.

Joey Adams

Due to the nature of our modern industrialized world, one of the fundamental difficulties we have with exercise today is that it is often seen as a separate aspect to our day-to-day life. As we have progressed from the Agricultural Age through to the Information Age, being active is no longer a part of most people's routine work. In places like Abkhasia, Hunza and other longevity hotspots, the vigorous daily activity of climbing up and down mountainsides, chasing one's herd or tilling the crops is part and parcel of everyday life—and one that is believed to be a key factor in their great health and longevity.

As most of us are more sedentary during the day, working on computers and the like, exercising becomes something that we see as separate to our working life. So we assign 20, 30 or 45 minutes, a few times a week—if we are lucky—to exercise. The consequence is that as the time we have available to exercise gets shorter, we've come to think that we have to increase our intensity level accordingly in order to get the same benefit. This is a bit like not having the time to cook a meal naturally in

---

a   Not everyone is designed to cultivate higher states of mind-body integration through physical exercise to the same degree. Just as each one of us is predisposed to succeeding in specific types of work, individually we are predisposed to develop such flow states in certain activities more than others. Some individuals will be more inclined to develop peak states in exercise, others more in vocational-type activities, and others in artistic endeavours such as music, painting, writing, sculpture or drama.

a conventional oven for twenty minutes, so zapping it in the microwave for three or four minutes. We think we are ending up with the same result, but unfortunately we aren't.

What this has bred is the myth of 'no pain no gain'. The prevailing wisdom today is that in order to receive benefits from exercise, whether in terms of cardiovascular benefits, muscular strength or flexibility, we have to push our bodies beyond our comfortable limit.

You may be familiar with this routine yourself. You get motivated to start an exercise program or join the local gym. On your first session you meet 'Jimmy the Gym Instructor'. Jimmy has 'accidentally' cut the sleeves of his shirt (revealing an impressive set of biceps), and when he is not looking at himself in the mirror, he gives you an initial program. Your immediate results are fantastic. Doing three or four sessions a week, you get fitter, stronger, and more energized. You feel a million dollars and all your friends comment on how much better you look. You are not sure whether to take this as a compliment, but as you are feeling so good, you do. Unfortunately, after an initial high your little fantasy world soon comes crashing down. Usually after about six to ten weeks, you come face to face with the dreaded '*Big P*'. This is not 'peak performance', 'perfect pecs' or the 'pleasure zone'. It is the killer of many a newly motivated exerciser: the big *PLATEAU*. As time wears on, you are told that you must increase the stress on your body to continue to see improvements. If you are one of the minority who have a specific goal, such as to drop a dress size for your wedding or to look good in your 'Borat mankini' in time for summer, you may be motivated to continue on. However, if you are one of the 80% of people who aren't naturally motivated to endure significant discomfort in your quest for health and fitness, after a period of time you will simply give up.

Unfortunately, to a large degree, we have been brainwashed into the athletes' way of health and fitness. We see our great athletes and revere them for their chiselled physiques and astounding feats of endurance, strength or speed—and assume that however they train must be the epitome of healthy exercise. However, looks can be deceiving. While athletes or finely-tuned sports stars might be super fit, they are often also 'super sick'. Have you ever noticed that before any big swim meet, a high number of swimmers are either fighting some sort of bug or have just recently got over one? Marathon runners, triathletes and other high-level athletes that train intensely for extended periods before reducing their training load prior to an event often have similar experiences. Continually pushing one's body beyond its comfortable limits can deplete the immune system and weaken the body generally. It also pays to have a look at athletes five, ten or twenty years after they stop competing. How many have arthritis? How many become stiff and inflexible? How many develop an aversion to exercise from all the years of discipline and stress? How many become sedentary, unfit and grossly overweight? We could also ask ourselves, 'If elite athletes are such supreme embodiments of health and fitness, why do the majority of them have to retire at 25 or 30 years of age?'

The point here is not to criticize athletes—the ideal of reaching for one's best is what life is all about. However, the reality is that the only individuals who tend to maintain a lifelong commitment to exercise based on 'no pain no gain' are those with strong, highly driven constitutions—the natural athletes, fitness instructors or ultra-determined types. Pushing oneself beyond one's limit might be the best current approach to achieve short-term athletic performance (though I believe there is a much better way to train even for elite sports performance), but this is not ideal for long-term health and wellbeing and has never been recommended in any of the long-established natural health sciences.

> Apart from the need for survival, exercise was traditionally associated with flow, dance, pleasure and joy. Today, the very thought of being active is often seen as an inconvenience or an undesirable necessity. Many of us need inspiration, discipline, a personal trainer or the distraction of music just to get us off the couch. These are signs that we have forgotten the natural wisdoms of exercise and lost our connection to the intrinsic joy of movement.

Towards more enlightened exercise in modern life

While zone states and higher states of awareness might be the ultimate purpose of exercise, the reality of our modern world is that just getting some more activity into our lives is a good start. By reminding ourselves of the natural wisdoms of exercise, we can increase both our motivation to exercise and the health benefits we receive from it.

The following points are designed to help you realign with these forgotten understandings. As most people have quite different propensities and desires when it comes to exercise, the points progress from ways to simply get more activity into one's day (points 1 and 2) through to ways to better unite mind, body and spirit (points 3 to 6). Simply choose whichever suits your own personal inclination.

1. FIND YOUR DANCE (OR AT LEAST ENJOY IT)

An hour of basketball feels like 15 minutes. An hour on a treadmill feels like a weekend in traffic school.

David Walters

We have become so obsessed with monitoring heart rates, measuring skin folds and counting repetitions, that many of us have forgotten the most important factor in any exercise. Physical activity is actually meant to be 'enjoyable'. Look at the average person, huffing and puffing on their daily run, gasping in a morning bootcamp, cringing in spin class or bemoaning the fact they need to go for a walk. How happy do they look? How many people who take part in 'fun runs' these days really have that much fun running? Just as we have lost the concept of using taste to help us determine the medicinal value of foods, to a large degree many people have lost sight of the fact that the enjoyment of exercise is just as important as the physical benefits. When we appreciate the inherent connection between our minds and bodies, a very important understanding presents itself. If we dislike doing a certain type of exercise, or feel stressed when doing it, we will not get the full benefits of that activity.

Let me repeat that another way.

You cannot actually receive the full physical benefits of exercise if you do not enjoy the activity you are doing.

As outlined in Wisdom One, the mind-body connection ensures that whatever we experience during exercise—joy, calmness, unbounded awareness, pain, frustration, impatience—produces a corresponding biochemistry in our body while we do it. If you dislike the type of exercise that you are doing, the chemistry of mental stress will be circulating throughout your body as you do it. While you will no doubt get the benefits of improved heart pumping, increased blood flow and respiratory efficiency, the inner chemical environment you create will simultaneously counteract some of those benefits. The low levels of regular exercise compliance in our Western world today are closely tied to the lack of enjoyment people associate with exercise. We say we don't have time to exercise, yet we have time to go to the movies, play computer games or sit in front of the TV. In many cases, the real reason we can't find time to exercise is that we don't enjoy it.

In most healthy, traditional cultures, beyond the high levels of physical activity performed as part of everyday life, people often participated in even more exercise. However, this wasn't for any other purpose than enjoyment. The Tarahumaras loved to run so they played games centered around running. The Hunzans have long played polo and the Okinawans gameball—a game similar to bowling. The common theme was 'play'. The game of life is meant to be just that, a game. Life is to be enjoyed. It is supposed to be fun, pleasurable, blissful. Movement of the physical body is designed to create that.

One of the most commonly cited benefits of exercise is the production of feel-good, relaxation-inducing endorphins. Endorphins are intimately tied to movement. Mother Nature has hard-wired us to move and in the same stroke gives us the experience of joy. Remember when you were a little boy or girl and just starting to walk or run. Do you remember how much fun it was? Today, many of us have forgotten the intrinsic joy of movement. Nowadays, people who hate going to the gym still go because 'gyms are where you go to get in shape'. Men who hate jogging continue to do it because 'that's what guys do'. Others exercise more out of compulsion than enjoyment because 'that's what doctors and experts say we should do'. In the quote at the beginning of this chapter, George Leonard reminds us that it's not just external results that are important when we do something, it's also how we feel on the inside while we do it. Do we dance?

Interestingly, dancing has been a part of basically every culture throughout history. Dancing is a perfect example of fun and pleasure through movement. Dancing promotes flow, and science tells us that dancing (and singing) connects our heart center to our brain center. It connects mind, body and soul. But I am not simply talking about the bridal waltz, ballroom, jazz, latin, rap or hip-hop dancing necessarily. These are just particular forms of an infinite number of dances. Dancing is anything that involves movement without us having to think about it. True dancing has no rules. When we have to dance a certain way, in a certain time, in a certain amount, our mind is often all that dances and we don't experience the joy. The only rule to dance is to move in a way that brings pleasure and joy. And for that there is a dance for everyone. For some it is the waltz, foxtrot or salsa. For others it's the thousand-year-old dances of their tribe. For some people it's running, swimming, hang-gliding, gardening, tennis or hiking through mountains. To move is to dance. So what's your dance?

How can you expand your perspective of exercise and find your dance? When you find what makes you dance, you will automatically lose weight, improve your heart health and get all the conventional benefits of exercise. In addition, you will have found yourself a life-long love affair that will ensure you never again have to be disciplined or motivated to exercise.

Finding your dance—Ideas to help

What do you enjoy, even love, that involves moving your body without having to measure heart rates, count repetitions or record calories burnt? What activities make you lose your sense of time and go beyond the endless analysis of modern exercise? If you could only do exercise you enjoyed, what would you do?

2. DON'T THINK 'EXERCISE' ... THINK ACTIVITY

Those who think they have no time for bodily exercise will sooner or later have to find time for illness.

Edward Stanley

In recent times, with the surge of obesity, diabetes, heart disease and many other modern-day illnesses, getting more exercise has understandably become a central focus. However, from the perspective of the natural laws of health, it is not necessarily structured exercise that is most important. A more accurate determinant, as supported by most research that looks at lifelong behaviors, is our overall day-to-day activity levels. One of the most consistent research findings among long-living populations is that regular physical activity is a natural part of their everyday lives.

Bama is a county in south-west China, which was recently named by the World Health Organization as a *'Hometown of Longevity'*. In Bama, the number of centenarians commonly matches that of the renowned Okinawa. Sally Beare gives an account of the lives of the Bama people in terms of their daily physical activity. 'Thanks to the mountains surrounding them on all four sides and the fact that they have no cars, the people of Bama get plenty of aerobic activity. The fact that they live 4,500 feet up in clean, oxygen-rich mountain air enhances the experience, of course. Couch potato syndrome is unknown in Bama—children have to climb the mountains to get to school, adults have to climb up and down them all day to tend their crops, and men enjoy hunting and archery even when they are in their eighties. The hard physical work involved in everyday life gives the people strong bones and muscles, including the heart muscle, and is no doubt an important factor behind their excellent health.'[4] (Most modern science suggests that it is the regularity rather the intensity of exercise that is most important for long-term health.)

Obviously our modern work and lifestyle demands make it largely impractical to follow the example of traditional cultures in terms of the volume of daily activity we perform. Fortunately, with the blessings of modern technology, most of us don't have this daily necessity. However, when we become so sedentary that it threatens our very lives—obesity, heart disease, diabetes etc are all significantly related to insufficient daily activity—it is clear we have lost our way. One of the simplest steps to address the problem of inactivity is to stop seeing exercise solely in its 'structured' form. The lesson from our healthy, long-living ancestors is that exercise does not need to be something that we allocate 30, 45 or 60 minutes to perform and do in a park or in a gym. It is not exercise per se that is essential but that we accumulate a certain amount of activity in our day-to-day lives. We need to expand our concept of exercise and appreciate that every little bit of movement counts. As this is what many health experts are already now advising, I do not wish to discuss it further here. However, if you are the type of person that is just not into exercise per se or has no interest in exploring the mind-body unifying approaches that follow, then as an absolute minimum walk or move your body for at least 45—60 minutes a day. (Suggestions for getting more activity into a busy Western lifestyle as well as further information on the popular 10,000 Steps program are included in the ebook).

Not long after completing an Honors degree in Exercise Physiology, I was introduced to a radically different philosophy of exercise through my studies in Maharishi Ayurveda. I learnt that the ancient Ayurvedic sages recommended that the principles of yoga should form the basis of all forms of daily exercise. While yoga has become extremely popular in the West as a way to reduce stress and integrate mind and body, when it comes to conventional exercise its principles are rarely discussed. However, Ayurveda suggests that by incorporating specific yoga practices into our everyday exercise routines, we can transform our experience from exertion to enjoyment, mind-body disintegration to mind-body integration and external stress to internal balance. The following three points relate to specific yoga principles that can both increase the benefits we derive from exercise as well as create a greater connection of mind, body and spirit.* They are the basis of what could be called 'enlightened exercise', and help fulfill the ultimate purpose of exercise as discussed earlier.

* It is acknowledged that the specific discussion and application of the principles of attention, nasal breathing and comfort to Western-style exercise, as well as many of the general principles and ideas discussed here, were first outlined by Dr. John Douillard in his 1994 book 'Body, Mind and Sport.' [5]

3. TAKE YOUR MIND WITH YOU

Where attention goes, energy flows.

Old Hawaiian Huna philosophy

Nearly every self-development or success coaching precept today advises us that '*what we put our attention on increases in our lives*'. It is one of the simplest yet most profound truths of our time. Ironically, when it comes to modern exercise, we generally do everything we can to do the exact opposite. We consciously try to take our attention away from whatever activity we are doing.

Think of most people walking or jogging at your local park. They will either be talking to a friend, talking on their mobile phone or listening to their iPod. At the gym, if they are not watching Oprah, Dr Phil or MTV, they are doing an exercise class where the music is so loud they can't even hear themselves think. When most of us exercise, our attention is directed outwards. The common reason for this is that we have been brainwashed into seeing exercise as something that is either boring or unpleasant. As such, we actively create ways to divert our minds from the boredom or discomfort that exercise entails.

Research shows that if we listen to music, we can exercise at higher intensities and have a reduced perception of pain. The current thinking is that this is a good thing. However the goal is not to endure greater discomfort, incur extra fatigue and disconnect our mind from our body. From the ancient understanding, the purpose of exercise is for us to enjoy the experience, rejuvenate our body and integrate it with our mind. We can only do this when we are listening to our body, not by listening to Oprah. Sorry Oprah.

Many years ago, I read of a very interesting study on muscle strength. A team of researchers got together three different groups and tested their baseline strength. The first group was instructed to lift a barbell of a certain weight for 20 repetitions, eight times a day for eight weeks. The second group was instructed not to do any weight training activities whatsoever for eight weeks. The third group was also instructed not to physically lift any weights for eight weeks. However, the individuals in this group were asked to lift the weighted barbell used by those in the first group once or twice, just to get a feel of its weight. They were then told to imagine or visualize lifting this barbell for 20 repetitions and to repeat this eight times a day for eight weeks. That is, they were to do the same as the first group but *mentally* rather than physically lift the weight.

After eight weeks, the individuals in the first group, who actually lifted the weights, had an increase in muscular strength of 30%. This was in line with expectations. The second group, or control group, who didn't do anything for eight weeks, as expected, had no improvement in muscle strength. Can you guess what results the third group, who merely visualized lifting the weights got? 0%? No, despite not actually lifting a weight, after eight weeks the average increase in muscular strength was ... 16%. This was just over half the increase of the group lifting the weights.

Interesting! How could this be? Well, it's actually not so astounding once we understand and appreciate that we are not merely physical machines, but rather mind-body beings. Although we usually think of physical activities as solely 'physical' events, for our bodies to be able to lift a weight, for example, the muscle fibers in our arms have to contract. They contract via messages from our nervous system. The messages our nervous system get are initiated via the central processing unit in our brain. Preceding our brain generating those impulses is a thought or desire within our mind to want to lift the weight.

So in any physical activity, we could say that approximately half of the performance relates to the physical action of body parts like our bones and muscles, and half to our mind and the intelligence connected to that.

After all, the diverse electrical, biochemical and hormonal products in any bodily process are just the concrete expressions of the mental activities through which we initiate them. What all this suggests is that for exercise to be maximally effective, it should be a mind and body activity.

The ancients suggest that if we want to significantly increase the results of our exercise, we should take our mind with us. When we are fully focused in exercise, we not only increase the effectiveness of what we are doing, but we are also less likely to find it boring. Additionally, we are better able to listen to our body's feedback as to what type and how much activity is best, as well as tuning in to any early signs of injury or fatigue.

When we put our attention on our body during exercise rather than on video hits, our iPod or Dr Phil, we make it a true mindbody integrating activity. Through inner attention, our exercise efficiency increases and we set the foundation for enjoying peak exercise experiences.

Mind-body exercise—Ideas to help

1. While you do not have to ditch your iPod or the cardio theatre every time you exercise, try it every now and then. Experiment with mind-body exercise. Occasionally go for a walk, a run, a swim or whatever you enjoy, and just have your complete, un-divided attention on your body. If swimming, notice your arms moving through the water. If jogging, feel the rhythm of your movement. Use your attention to deepen your breathing and re-lax your muscles.

2. To supercharge your mind-body awareness, try exercising with your eyes closed for brief periods. This works great with activities such as weight training, exercise-bike cycling, machine rowing and even swimming if you are away from walls and other swim-mers. I don't recommend it quite so enthusiastically while running on treadmills, walking on busy roads or cycling near cliffs—lol!

3. When doing yoga or any activity involving stretching your body, focus fully on the specific muscles you are stretching. Actually feel the stretch and be intimately aware of the specific point where the muscle fibers begin to tense up and become restricted. Notice how by focusing the power of your attention at this point, you can dissolve some of the tension or tightness in the muscles and promote greater flexibility.

4. Sports 'play': If you play sports, remember when you were a little kid—before you knew about scores or what the right technique was? Do you remember playing just for the absolute fun of it? There was no right or wrong, good or bad, win or lose. There was just 'play'. If you still play a sport, every now and then take your attention away from any external factors and instead focus on the intrinsic enjoyment of the actual movement, flow or the game itself. Just play as you did when you were a little boy or girl. Forget the score. Forget about 'the right way' to hold the club or swing the racquet and just 'play'.

4. BREATHE LIKE THE YOGIS

Its very simplicity keeps thousands from seriously considering it, while they spend fortunes in seeking health through complicated and expensive systems .... Verily the stone which the builders reject is the real cornerstone of the Temple of Health.

Yogi Ramacharaka on proper breathing

What is arguably the simplest and most profound way of promoting exercise-high experiences is also the one that is most commonly overlooked. It is that of breathing. While we spend countless amounts of time and energy on the latest heart rate monitors, lifting techniques, running gear and nice-looking leotards (at least I do), one of the most fundamental aspects of effective mind-body exercise—how to breathe properly—is almost never taught.

Now you might think that breathing is an entirely natural phenomenon, so how on earth could breathing be a forgotten wisdom of exercise? In short, it is because there are two ways we can breathe. The first is how most people breathe. This method initiates the body's stress response and increases the likelihood of early fatigue, lightheadedness and muscle soreness. The second way of breathing is how Mother Nature designed us to breathe and can help transport our experience of exercise to wondrous new heights. So profound are the benefits of simply breathing properly that many Oriental philosophies suggest that it has the power to prevent sickness, eliminate illness and even enliven dormant spiritual powers. When combined with the power of our attention, the Yogi Masters taught that the way we breathe can be considered a complete mind-body exercise in itself. The great kung fu masters credit much of their ability to perform what are often considered superhuman feats of strength and endurance to the ability to control their breathing.

Unfortunately, with the loss of such wisdom, we Westerners have become inefficient, sickly breathers. The most common way 90% of us breathe during any reasonable level of exertion (more than a leisurely walk), is via upper-chest mouth breathing. When we employ shallow mouth breathing, we draw most of the air into our upper lungs, where we have far less blood supply. The air that enters our lungs also tends to be dry, cold and full of impurities. This is because our mouths have no humidifying, heating or filtering mechanisms. Such breathing triggers our body's sympathetic nervous system, or what is more commonly known as our *'fight-or-flight' response*. The fight-or-flight response is directly associated with increased heart rates, breath rates, physical tension, stress hormones and asthmatic reactions. With this style of functioning, our metabolic activity is also far less efficient. We burn relatively more carbohydrates, our short-term fuel source, rather than fat, our longer-term fuel source. Due to the inefficient metabolism it promotes, mouth breathing can also indirectly increase fatigue, free radical damage and lactic acid levels. Lactic acid is related to the heavy feeling you might experience in your muscles during more vigorous exercise.

As our body's survival response mechanism, mouth breathing is geared for short-term, stressful situations where we need a quick burst of oxygen to our muscles. In a true survival situation this is wonderful, even life-saving. However, oxygen does not go directly to our brain when we mouth breathe. This reduces the level of mind-body connection we experience and promotes a far greater likelihood of lightheadedness, upper respiratory tract infections and general discomfort.

Nature's way to optimal breathing

Man should no more breathe through his mouth than he would attempt to take food in through his nose.

Yogi Ramacharaka

If you have ever done yoga, pilates, tai chi or other Eastern-based exercise, you will know that the way Mother Nature designed us to breathe is via deep, diaphragmatic nasal breathing. While we will give a quick overview here, for a full account see Yogi Ramacharaka's magnificent book *'Science of Breath'*.[6]

Despite the fact that many people breathe through their mouths for large parts of the day without even being aware of it, we were designed to breathe through our noses. When we breathe with our mouth closed (harder for some I know), our little nasal hairs capture and prevent any unwanted airborne particles from entering our lungs. The blood-rich membranes and thick mucous linings of our nasal cavities warm and moisten the air. This not only ensures the air doesn't shock the sensitive inner tissues and set off our body's fight-or-flight response, it also establishes the most conducive conditions for oxygen transfer in our lungs. Our lungs do not like dry air, which is partly why mouth breathing is more closely associated with asthma, particularly exercise-induced asthma.

As we naturally breathe more deeply and slowly through the nose, our diaphragm has time to contract fully. In what Yogis call *'low breathing'*, the nasal breath is as if drawn deep into the belly. This creates a vacuum-like sucking of the air deep into our lungs where it meets with a most abundant blood supply. With upper-chest mouth breathing, the air floods in so quickly it goes mainly to the upper portions of our lungs where there is far less blood supply. In the West we think of oxygen as the critical component of the air we breathe. This is true on the gross physical level of the body. However, just as with the food we eat, on a deeper level, the ancients understood that is the subtle life-force or prana that is the key ingredient. While oxygen nourishes our blood and muscles, it is prana that fundamentally nourishes our mind and nervous system. As opposed to mouth breathing, when we nasal breathe, the life-force energy is brought directly into our brain stem via our receptors for smell. This instantaneously enlivens our entire brain and nervous system.

Most importantly, when we nasal breathe we heighten the communication between the left and right hemispheres of our brain and holistically integrate mind and body. This results in improved focus and clarity of mind, enhanced decision-making and greater psychological resilience. Deep nasal breathing also eliminates the possibility of over-breathing or over-ventilation, which some science now links to increased aging. One possibility as to why people who regularly meditate or do yoga-related practices commonly live healthier, longer lives is that they have significantly lower oxygen intakes and thus subject themselves to less free radical damage. (Most free radicals are oxygen-based.) The fact that nasal breathing is associated with our body's relaxation response rather than our stress response would also help. This is why many natural health sciences promote proper breathing to effectively treat stress-based conditions such as anxiety, insomnia and asthma.

Proper breathing—exercise for the 'internal organs'

Aerobic exercise is commonly associated with keeping our heart and lungs healthy, and resistance training for strengthening our muscles and bones. Unfortunately, what we often overlook in our Western view of exercise is exercising our vital internal organs. In many health magazines today, a ripped sixpack, toned arms and sexy legs are often flaunted as the epitome of being fit and healthy. However, the Eastern masters tell us that these aren't particularly important if our kidneys are functioning at half capacity, our liver is clogged or our bowels are blocked. The ancients understood that the health of our internal organs—our heart, liver, spleen, kidneys, intestines—is far more important than having a washboard stomach, bulging biceps or a taut butt. They also knew that the way to keep these organs healthy was through exercise—internal exercise. Specific yoga postures known as 'asanas' and deep, diaphragmatic breathing were routinely recommended as they were both understood to softly massage, tone and increase blood flow to our vital internal organs. Both practices also promote the efficient elimination of waste products from the body while simultaneously exercising the rib cage and upper spine to prevent them becoming stiff and inflexible. Combined, they represent a key component of the ancient formula for maintaining peak health and inner balance.

By breathing the way the great yogis have taught, through the nose and fully engaging the diaphragm, we maximally eliminate impurities and increase our energy, vitality and resistance to fatigue. We also stimulate our body's relaxation response to slow our heart rate, soften our breath, relax our muscles, and create a settled yet heightened state of mind-body connectedness.

If you want to promote the highest level of mind-body health, don't just eat well, breathe well.

Do it now breathing exercise

Correct breathing that can improve your quality of life, help combat the effects of aging and provide the foundation for your most effective exercise is based on what the yogis call 'Yogi complete breathing.'

Right now, sit upright, close your eyes, put your hands on your abdomen and take your awareness to your breathing. Breathe slowly and comfortably through your nose. With each inhalation, rather than raising your shoulders to fill your upper chest, allow your abdomen to relax and feel as if you are breathing deep into your lower abdomen. Feel your diaphragm (the muscle just under your rib cage) massaging your abdominal organs and notice your abdomen begin to rise slightly. As your abdomen comfortably finishes its expansion, extend your inhaling breath to first fill your middle chest and then your upper chest. Allow these areas, including your whole rib cage, to expand. Don't try to extend the duration of your inhalation unnaturally or hold your breath. Just keep it natural and comfortable.

For the first few breaths, notice the momentary pause between the end of the 'in' breath and the start of the 'out' breath. Like the in and out flow of tides and seasons, this junction point between the inflowing and outflowing breath is representative of the natural cycles of life. Just being aware of the gap between your breaths—the ebb and flow of your breathing—is a powerful way to reconnect your body with the universal rhythms of Mother Nature.

Taking your attention to your abdominal area for a few more breaths, notice how you can eliminate more air by contracting your abdominal muscles slightly as you exhale—also through your nose. After these breaths, just exhale naturally and, using your attention, allow the exhalation to extend as long as is comfortable. Feel the old, impure air being released from your body as you pave the way for a new, fresh batch of life-giving oxygen and prana to enter.

Spend a minute or two breathing this way now and practice it at least a couple of times a day. Good times may include while driving, watching TV or sitting in a seminar. It can also be used as a stand-alone remedy when feeling stressed or anxious, experiencing tension headaches, or if unable to sleep at night due to an over-excited or restless mind.

NOTE: Consciously utilizing your abdominal muscles during exhalation can be particularly effective when experiencing stress or tension or in the recovery portions of higher-intensity exercise. However, it need not be employed during exercise itself. In general daily activity and most exercise, do not try to force or control your breathing in any way. Keep it as natural and effortless as possible.

Nasal breathing in exercise

Although many people learn to breathe properly when doing yoga, pilates, tai chi or similar stress management classes, in the case of aerobic exercise most of us don't even consider it. However, the same deep, relaxed nasal breathing outlined above is how we are meant to breathe at even the highest levels of exercise. All the problems associated with mouth breathing, such as increased physical tension, inefficient metabolic functioning and mind-body disconnection, are all significantly exacerbated during higher levels of activity, e.g. exercise. By employing Mother Nature's way of breathing, as opposed to the stress-based mouth breathing that most people employ, you can transform your experience of exercise.

Nasal breathing during exercise:

- makes the body more relaxed and reduces physical tension
- improves respiratory (breathing) efficiency
- reduces fight-or-flight activation and slows heart rate
- delivers oxygen directly to the brain, heightening connection of mind and body
- eliminates light-headedness or shortness of breath
- significantly reduces asthmatic reactions / exercise-induced asthma
- increases endurance and resistance to fatigue over time
- promotes a higher proportion of fat rather than carbohydrate metabolism
- indirectly reduces free radical damage and muscle soreness via effects on metabolism
- reduces incidence of colds, sinus congestion, upper respiratory infections and even sleep apnea
- makes it more enjoyable (exercising feels better) and increases the likelihood of having *'peak experiences'* or *'flow states.'*

Real life nasal breathing examples

At this moment, you may be thinking that you couldn't possibly get enough air in through your nose when exercising. As this is a common response, and although we are focused on everyday health and wellbeing here, I thought to share a couple of examples of how this breathing technique has been used even in the sporting arena to convince you that everyone can and should breathe this way during exercise.

I first learnt about employing nasal breathing in exercise back in 1994. I was still playing AFL football at the time and it was mid-season. While it was difficult to incorporate immediately, by the pre-season (the hardest training phase of the year) of 1995 I was able to complete about 90% of all training while breathing nasally. The only time that I couldn't maintain nasal breathing was during flat out, high intensity activities such as 50m sprint repetitions, maximum weight training lifts or one-on-one competitive drills. The only other time was when I would burst out laughing at my teammate's attempts to nasal breathe during 400m sprints without any prior practice—that was a good laugh! This is not to suggest that I found the training easy just by breathing differently. It was by no means enjoyable. However, in comparison to the previous years' training, the difference I experienced in terms of subjective pain, time to fatigue, and particularly the reduced time for recovery following sessions, was dramatic. Although I was still pushing myself, I didn't feel the usual exhaustion after sessions. I would feel better the next day and felt generally fresher throughout the entire season. (Too bad it couldn't help the other deficiencies in my game!)

After convincing myself that this way of breathing was a far more intelligent way to go, I started teaching it to others. Results from other AFL footballers, national league netballers and a colleague who subsequently taught it to some Olympic-level athletes showed the benefits were universal. If people did not have any structural problems, e.g. a severely deviated septum (nose bone), nasal breathing comfortably at any decent level of exertion was not a problem. The only obstacle was that people had to be willing to persist through the first few weeks of reduced performance and possible breathing difficulties.

One of the best examples I saw was with a colleague and friend, Murray Beveridge. Murray was a professional middle distance runner. Middle distance races such as the 800 meters are arguably the most challenging in terms of being able to complete them while maintaining nasal breathing. Murray was at the elite level. He was state level and ran at many high-level competitions including National Championships. When I explained the benefits of using nasal breathing, Murray really liked it and was very conscientious in his efforts to integrate this method of breathing into his training and competition regime.

The benefits seemed to accumulate steadily each and every month. Within a two-month period, he found that his heart rate for his regular

5km run dropped from 157 to 148bpm. He also cut his time by more than two minutes—an incredible improvement. He attributed all this to changing and committing himself to nasal breathing. Being a professional athlete, Murray was training every day. So within just a few months, he became quite proficient as a nasal breather. After about six months, he was actually able to introduce some nasal breathing into his competitive races. Less than a year after starting to nasal breathe, Murray won the Stawell Gift 800m handicap race. The Stawell Gift, held over Easter in country Victoria each year, is the best known event for handicap racing throughout Australia. However, the part I love the most was when Murray explained one day that he was becoming known as a bit of a freak around the race meeting circuit. You see, the most common sight at the end of races, particularly 800m races, is that of athletes straining, red-faced and with mouths wide open trying to gulp down every last ounce of air. Murray, however, became such an effective nasal breather that at the end of his races he was still breathing through his nose. His mouth was completely shut. The image of him coming to the finish line, seemingly not even breathing, became a topic of much interest among spectators. He remarked, 'People would come up to me after races and ask me what was going on. They would say, "You weren't even breathing". Their reaction was hilarious. I almost felt like a bit of a freak show.'

These examples, as well as countless others, show us that if athletes can nasal breathe at high performance levels then we should be able do it in lower level activities for our everyday health and wellness. The key is to simply start integrating nose breathing into exercise gradually. The first few weeks can be a little frustrating as the airways are usually not very well conditioned due to previous neglect, i.e. improper breathing, but be patient.

Nasal breathing in exercise—Ideas to help

Step 1: Practice nasal breathing without activity

Before you try to integrate nasal breathing into your normal exercise sessions, take some mini-steps. At every opportunity, practice comfortable, full-capacity breathing while you are in a completely rested state. As mentioned, this might include while driving, watching TV, working (daydreaming) at your desk and even while sitting on the toilet—'things' move better the more relaxed you are!

This will help open up your sinus channels and condition your lungs, diaphragm and rib cage to more comfortably nasal breathe once you start exercising.

Step 2: Nasal breathe during light daily activities

Before using nasal breathing in high-level exercise, first condition your respiratory system with low-level daily activities. Starting on an exercise bike is ideal as it is highly controlled and allows a low level of activity while having full attention on your breathing. Other possibilities include walking around your home, walking to work and walking your dog.

Step 3: Nasal breathe in warm-ups, cool-downs and low-level exercise

When you start employing nasal breathing in your exercise sessions, start at low intensities first. If you don't want to reduce your exercise level too much while waiting for your breathing to become more efficient—maybe you are exercising with others or are involved in a team sport—simply focus on diaphragmatic nasal breathing during warm-ups and cool-downs, and breathe however is comfortable during the main activity portion.

NOTE: If you are going to exercise beyond your comfort zone (see Point 5), warm-ups and cool-downs are highly recommended to minimize any adverse effects.

> *Step 4: Nasal breathe throughout your whole exercise session*
>
> As you become more conditioned to nasal breathing, use it as is comfortable throughout all of your exercise sessions. If you play a sport that requires you to go beyond your comfortable nasal breathing limit, focus on coming back to your breathing during any rest or recovery periods, e.g. in between points during tennis, when the ball goes out of play in soccer, or during free throws or substitutions in basketball.

Follow your nose

In Ayurveda, our ability to nasal breathe is said to determine how much and how quickly we are supposed to exercise. That is, our breathing dictates our optimal exercise intensity and duration.

With this in mind, if you are exercising purely for health and balance purposes, once you have established a moderate level of nasal breathing proficiency, begin tuning in to your breathing to help determine your ideal exercise pace. Perform your chosen activity to a level where you can breathe through your nose in a comfortable, relaxed way. If your breathing becomes strained or loses its comfortable rhythm, reduce your exercise level until it again feels easy and comfortable. At higher levels of activity, the depth and rate of your breathing may initially increase slightly, but it should still be completely relaxed and comfortable. Assuming a minimum of three to four exercise sessions a week, within four to twelve weeks you should be able to perform whatever level of activity you could previously while nasal breathing. This can include high level aerobic exercise, should you choose to do it.

At a seminar in Hobart (Australia) in 2007, a gentleman came up to me in the morning tea break to tell me that he had been using nasal breathing as his exercise intensity barometer all his life. He told me how he really enjoyed exercise when he breathed through his nose. However, whenever he had to push himself to the point of finding it difficult to nasal breathe, it 'just didn't feel right'. He explained how his whole body would react once he started mouth breathing, and that he just couldn't understand why anyone would exercise this way. I wholeheartedly agreed.

> The more you can condition yourself to maintain comfortable nasal breathing while exercising, the more you train your body to integrate this more efficient, high-performance state into your everyday activities.
>
> Whether you are sleeping, doing your weekly yoga class or are involved in a high stress situation, this more resilient inner functioning will enable you to do it more effectively.

Breathing to supercharge stretching and weight training

In considering the healthiest people to have lived, it is apparent that it is not just living a long time that is important. Living with energy, vitality and inner contentment is the real beauty. In this regard, both the practice of yoga and the martial arts are commonly found among individuals who have exemplified exceptional inner and outer health. From the remarkably robust Shaolin monks to age-defying yoga masters, practices that unite the inner and outer body are often found at the basis of a healthy life. In many forms of yoga and the martial arts, it is the power of attention and breathing that accomplished practitioners combine to supercharge their results.

Yoga masters are known to be able to store prana or life-force energy in their bodies, and even channel it to particular organs, through the focus of their attention. By combining proper breathing with the power of attention, it is said that they can direct the all-important life-force to strengthen or even heal a poorly functioning heart, liver, spleen or kidney. Kung fu students are taught focused exhalation breathing techniques that quickly release bodily tension to add incredible power to their kicks, punches and blocks. The seemingly amazing feats of certain martial arts practitioners do not come from sheer physical strength but also from the strength of their mind's attention and the power of their breathing.

Focusing on our breathing during weight training, body circuit training or flexibility stretching can similarly enhance our results. Traditionally, the inhaled breath is associated with drawing the life-force into the body, and the exhaled breath is associated with releasing energy and tension from the body. As such, in weight training or lifting exercises, a simple rule to remember is the *'E' Rule*. Whenever you are doing the exertion phase, exhale. On any recovery or resting phase, inhale. For example, if you are lifting weights above your head, breathe out while pushing the weight up and breathe in while bringing the weight down. In a chin-up, breathe out while lifting yourself up and breathe in while lowering yourself down.

To enhance the mind-body integration aspect of weight training, some people also coordinate the speed of their repetitions with the comfortable rhythm of their breath. That is, they lift the weight in time with their exhalation and lower the weight in time with their inhalation. This creates a nice connection between mind, body and breathing and is often enjoyed by those who already practice yoga or simply like a bit more refinement to the conventional way of lifting weights. Generally, it is best to breathe both in and out through the nose, especially for aerobic exercise or moderate, circuit-type routines. If you are lifting heavier weights with lower repetitions, breathe in through your nose and out through your mouth if it is more comfortable.

When performing stretching exercises, inhale while holding your mind's attention at the comfortable point of the stretch. You may even like to visualize the healing breath coming into the muscle or muscle group you are stretching. During exhalation, let the muscle or muscle group relax and release any tension. If it does, gently extend into a deeper stretch during this exhalation phase.

Try it now stretching exercise

Sit on the floor with your left leg bent, so that the sole of your foot is on the inside of your right knee. Bend forward at the hips to stretch your hands towards your toes. This is a common lower back and hamstring stretch that most of us normally do with minimal attention or focus on our breathing.

Having your full attention on your right hamstrings (the muscles at the back of the thigh), bend forward until you get to the point where you cannot comfortably stretch any further. There should be no pain, just some gentle resistance. Pause at this point and bring your attention to your breathing. As you breathe in, mentally direct the energy and power of your breath into your hamstring muscles, particularly to any areas of tightness. Feel the power of your breath move into the muscles and help dissolve any tension. As you exhale, allow your hamstrings and your body generally to let go of any tightness.

NOTE: Only increase your stretch if your muscles relax naturally. Do not try to force the stretch with the will of your mind. You will notice that the more you push your muscles to stretch, the more they will resist. This is symbolic of everything in the natural world and a good reminder that what is most evolutionary and health-promoting comes not from forcing but from allowing.

Even apart from exercise, diaphragmatic nasal breathing is a pillar of health and happiness. Look to incorporate it into all your daily activities, and use exercise as a way to condition your breathing efficiency to new heights. During exercise, do not force, control or try to manipulate your breathing in any way. Don't try to excessively deepen your breathing or consciously extend its duration. Just be conscious of breathing comfortably through your nose. Breathe from your belly rather than your chest or shoulders, and simply allow your breath to find its own comfortable depth and rhythm. Keep it natural and easy and you will enjoy a whole new, more enjoyable experience of exercise.

> By employing deep nasal breathing during aerobic exercise, you will maximize your exercise efficiency and open up the possibility of enjoying heightened states of integration and flow.
>
> In such 'peak states', you may feel as if you are hardly breathing at all. This is a perfect reminder of Mother Nature's eternal recipe for success.
>
> Breathe less, achieve more.

5. STAY 'IN' YOUR COMFORT ZONE

Nature does not hurry, yet everything is accomplished.

Lao Tzu

Despite the almost universal credo that we have to work hard and 'get out of our comfort zones' to achieve success in life, this was not always considered the height of wisdom. Mother Nature never 'works hard'. She works by the principle of least effort. The changing of the seasons, the cycles of day and night and the falling of rain all occur as part of an effortless flow. Karl Barth once commented on the joys of listening to Mozart. 'Mozart's music always sounds unburdened, effortless, and light. This is why it unburdens, releases, and liberates us.' Similarly, it is only when we do things, including exercise, in ways that are unburdened, effortless and light that we truly experience release and liberation.

Wise teachers throughout time have contended that Mother Nature always guides us to what is best for our life and our success. On the one hand there is the feeling of ease, enjoyment, joy, exhilaration, bliss and '*being totally in the moment*'. On the other hand there is the experience of strain, effort, fatigue, and the feeling of being disconnected or '*out of sync*'. The experience of ease, enjoyment and comfort is our way of knowing that what we are doing is appropriate. Pain, exhaustion or discomfort are signs that something is not right. Stop! Wrong way! Go back! They are not signals that we are getting somewhere worthwhile and need to push on through the pain barrier. While working hard, in the sense of putting a certain amount of time, energy and focus into a job or relationship, is critical for our success, the concept of needing to push or strain is not a part of Mother Nature's eternal success formula. Exercise is no different.

In the Tarahumara Indian culture, where running is based on ease and enjoyment rather than 'no pain no gain', the older one gets, the better a runner one becomes. The grandfathers are esteemed as the best athletes. How can this be? It seems that without years of accumulating stress and strain from pushing themselves beyond their comfortable limits, their bodies become more efficient and thus move more effortlessly. Zone states, the ultimate experiences any exercise enthusiast can enjoy, are associated with effortlessness and ease, not stress and strain. Throughout the history of elite sports, a common experience from world record-breaking, gold medal-winning, or personal best-setting athletes is that their greatest performances were often the most effortless and enjoyable of their careers. The media rush up to them saying, 'What a performance, you must have worked so hard'. The athlete replies along the lines of, 'It's funny you know, I just felt really comfortable out there. I wasn't straining at all. I got into this really nice rhythm and it all just flowed. It's like my legs weren't even touching the ground. I felt like I could have kept going all day'.

When we think of our own most enjoyable experiences, whether they be in sport, work, an artistic endeavour, a hobby or a relationship, all are more likely to have the qualities of ease, effortlessness and flow rather than stress, struggle and hard work. With this in mind, it seems odd that burdening ourselves with stress and discomfort could in any way help us attain the ultimate exercise benefits. In fact, according to ancient wisdom, the final pillar for making exercise most effective is to do the exact opposite of what we are commonly told. Instead of getting out of our comfort zone, the ancients tell us that the highest wisdom is to stay 'in' our comfort zone.

Your dynamic comfort zone

In suggesting that exercising only to the point of comfort is ideal for our mind-body health, this does not imply that we should only exercise at very low levels. We know that being a couch potato is disastrous for our health. Similarly, regularly exercising beyond our body's comfortable limits increases our risk of injury, illness and in some cases even sudden death. However, like *'the middle way'* that the Buddha taught, the middle of the two extremes of exercise is where the ancients declared our ideal exercise zone to be.

In the 6000-year-old records of Ayurveda, it is specifically recommended that exercise be performed at 50% of our capacity. That's right, just 50%. While such a figure sounds extremely low to most people, at 50% capacity we have adequate oxygen to meet our energy requirements. At this level, our bodies burn fat as their predominant fuel and generate minimal waste products in the muscles. In Ayurveda, this is also known as the intensity where we experience maximum mind-body integration and set the foundation for peak exercise experiences. In short, we get the many benefits of exercise while optimizing our subjective enjoyment. Once we go beyond 50% of our capacity, we initiate the body's fight-or-flight response and produce energy far less efficiently. This inevitably comes with a corresponding feeling of heaviness, muscle soreness, fatigue, reduced enjoyment, and a diminished sense of mind-body unification—the key goal of exercise.

> At 50% of exercise capacity, we get all the benefits of exercise—including a natural shower of 'feel good' endorphins—without strain or discomfort.
>
> By exercising in our comfort zone, we maximally connect mind and body, and experience the joy of exercise rather than the pain of exercise.

Knowing where your 'comfort zone' is

If you like measuring your heart rate while you exercise, the most accurate correlation of 50% capacity is approximately 60% of your maximum heart rate. However, I generally recommend against monitoring heart rates when exercising at this level. This is not to contradict athletes, fitness advisors or personal trainers who use them. We are simply talking about two distinctly different approaches here. As the whole purpose of yoga-styled exercise is to enjoy the experience and to connect mind and body (yoga literally means 'to yoke' or 'unite'), we don't want to divert our attention away from our body and have our awareness governed by a wristwatch.

Heart rate monitors can help some people get motivated to exercise and show fitness improvements, which is obviously good. However, they can reinforce the belief that 'science' is more reliable than our body's own intelligence. We think the heart rate monitor or the latest scientific recommendation of exercise intensity is God, and we forget to tune in to our body's infinite inner wisdom. Eventually we end up like robots, focused on heart rates, calories burnt or exercise time endured, and overlook the fact that our bodies have their own perfect, in-built intensity monitor. It's called enjoyment. Do we really need some external digital device beeping at us to tell us we are exercising too hard? Surely gasping like a two-pack-a-day chain smoker and wondering 'when is this all going to end?' should tell us that. The best way to assess your ideal (50%) exercise intensity is to simply tune in and LISTEN! Like life, exercise is much simpler than we make it. In its infinite wisdom, your body will correlate all the innumerable factors affecting it at any one time and tell you whether your exercise level is appropriate via the experience of comfort or discomfort. Exercise comfort means maximal efficiency, motivation and long-term effectiveness. Discomfort or pain equates to compromised motivation, mind-body disconnection and short-term fitness gains, often at the expense of long-term health. As mentioned, this exercise approach can be fine for individuals with strong, highly driven constitutions—the natural athletes, fitness instructors or highly determined types—but it is not ideal for most people.

The next time you exercise, try the following. Start your activity at a very low level and gradually build up your exercise pace—or weight resistance etc. While tuning in to your body, gauge your overall comfort level and assess the suitability of your exercise according to feeling:

1. physically *lighter*
2. more *energized*
3. more *connected* in mind and body

If you feel the opposite of any of these—maybe your legs or arms start to feel heavy, your breathing becomes strained, or you experience some mental disconnection—just reduce your pace or exercise load. The key to enjoying exercise that will unify your mind and body and motivate you to do it time and again is to stay below this level of discomfort. That is to stay 'in' your comfort zone. Rather than trying to go faster, which you could do temporarily by going into 'stress mode', get used to staying at the upper limit of your comfort zone. Notice how exercising at this level makes you feel lighter, more energized and more centered. If you are just after general health benefits, your exercise will also be maximally enjoyable. If you are more into performance improvement then, as your body becomes more efficient, it will gradually learn to perform at higher levels of efficiency. You will gradually go faster based on improved efficiency rather than on adrenaline.

Mark is a friend of mine who learnt these principles some years ago. I asked him to recount the typical experiences he has when he goes swimming. He responded as follows:

> It's funny, although I'm still reasonably fit, I always start off in the slow lane. For the first few minutes I almost sink I'm going so slow. Even some of the golden oldies give me dirty looks (and often a sly elbow) as they have to swim past me. However, if I take it super easy to begin with, my body gradually becomes lighter and looser. After ten minutes I'm usually into a nice cruisy swim and soon it's me who's banging up against the notoriously slow swimmers in front—every public swimming pool has them! I find the key at this stage is just to keep things easy. When I do this, the time seems to fly and I can really enjoy the actual process of gliding through the water. If I'm patient enough and restrain myself from wanting to swim faster, often after twenty minutes I'm swimming at quite a good speed, commonly having to progress to the fast lane. However, even at this pace I'm not gasping for air or feeling that my arms or legs are tired or heavy. I'm still cruising and often feel like I could keep going all day. Usually at the end I like to push it for the last few hundred meters. Even then, while it's not entirely effortless, I feel the exhilaration without the normal level of strain and discomfort I used to experience when I went hard right from the start. I love it.

If you are used to pushing yourself to your limits or feel guilty unless you punish yourself to the point of exhaustion, you may initially find exercising in your comfort zone quite frustrating. However, just as removing dirt from the tracks of a train allows the train to run faster with less power, the more stress and inefficiency (friction) you remove from your body, the more quickly it can move with less effort. Exercising this way will also protect you from injury, motivate you to exercise more often, and promote the optimal conditions for you to experience an exercise high.

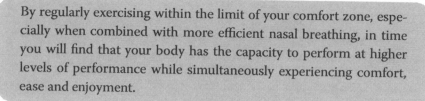

By regularly exercising within the limit of your comfort zone, especially when combined with more efficient nasal breathing, in time you will find that your body has the capacity to perform at higher levels of performance while simultaneously experiencing comfort, ease and enjoyment.

Staying in your comfort zone—Ideas to help

1. Recondition your thinking to see exercise as a completely enjoyable and pleasurable activity.
2. Exercise according to the experience of comfort and ease rather than stress and discomfort. Exercise at the highest level you can while still feeling comfortable. Don't push yourself to go faster. Let improved efficiency increase your performance rather than increased effort or strain.
3. If you play a sport, or just like the exhilaration of pushing yourself beyond your comfortable limit every now and then, that's fine. In such cases, however, look to do an extended warm-up where you spend five to fifteen minutes slowly building up to higher levels of performance. Such a graded build-up, where you establish a foundation of comfort, ease and efficient breathing, will at least minimize any detrimental effects and allow some level of mind-body connection to be integrated into your activity.

6. EXERCISE FOR TRANSCENDENCE

The human individual, ultimately, is spirit, and can participate to some extent in the larger consciousness even while embodied in flesh.

George Leonard[7]

This section will not be for everyone, but has been included briefly for those who want to explore the possibilities of higher levels of exercise experience.

The Tarahumara Indians, mentioned at the beginning of this chapter, have races with neighboring tribes that can go for days. The races usually consist of tribes running together kicking a small ball. If a tribe loses their ball, they lose the race. Interestingly, the ball serves not just as an integral part of the race but as a central focus for the runner's attention. Combining the physical feat of long-distance running with the constant mental demands of focusing on the ball creates a mind-body integration similar to meditation—an 'active meditation' as it were. Thus, for these tribes, the experience of running for hours or days on end is not mindnumbingly boring, but can become an experience of almost spiritual significance. Other forms of exercise can bring similar results. As George Leonard explains, 'The rhythmic, repetitive movements of the body and the steady flow of visual stimuli are well constituted to induce visions and reveal mysteries.'[8]

> When we combine physical exercise with something that entrains our mental functioning, we too can experience 'mystical' moments of timelessness and transcendence.

Exercise as an active meditation

If you ever get sick of just going to the gym or enduring some form of structured exercise, try the following. Think of exercise as an active meditation. As when meditating, try to find a location that is relatively quiet and free from distractions. To begin with, look to engage in a consistently repetitive type activity where you can easily govern your exercise pace. Good examples are walking, jogging, cycling, rowing, kayaking or swimming. In most forms of meditation, something is used to focus the mind's attention and promote mind-body integration, such as one's breathing or a mantra. Similarly, doing an activity of a consistent, repetitive nature will allow you to better connect your mind and body to promote the highest degree of union.

Focusing on the natural rhythm of your breathing is a great way to begin integrating your mind and body. By taking your attention to your breathing, you not only maximize its efficiency—'*where attention goes, energy flows*'—but internalize the whole process of exercise. This automatically reduces external distractions. After a very gradual warmup, establish a nice, comfortable pace using deep, diaphragmatic nasal breathing. At this point, simply direct your attention to the repetitive nature of your breath: in, out, in out, in, out. Do not to try to control your breathing in any way. Do not try to make it deeper or longer. Do not even forcibly hold your attention on the repetitive nature of your breathing. Just be *aware* of it. Simply enjoy the experience of comfort and notice your breathing. If at any point you become aware that your attention has been drawn away, for example you start thinking about what you are doing on the weekend or how strange you might look by enjoying your exercise, just comfortably bring your awareness back to the repetitive nature of your breath.

Once you find your breathing is completely easy and your mind's attention is remaining comfortably on your breathing without distraction, gradually let your awareness expand outwards to the repetitive nature of the activity itself. If you are jogging, take your attention to your legs or your feet as they hit the ground. If swimming, focus on your arms or your hands as they glide through the water. If kayaking, it might be the alternating pulling of the paddle through the water. Finally, after having your attention on the rhythmic nature of the activity itself for a while, allow your awareness to go to the overall flow of the activity or movement. Gradually allow your awareness to expand and almost feel yourself 'witnessing' your body doing the activity. It might feel as if you are on autopilot or that you are almost outside your body looking in. Note, however, that you are not trying to create an out-of-body experience. You actually want to have an 'in-your-body' experience.

The last stage before slipping into the flow state of exercise involves an expanded state of awareness. Having your attention on your feet hitting the ground, your arms pushing through the water or on your breathing helps direct your mind inward and away from external distractions—that is, you zone in. Ultimately, however, you do not want to direct your attention in any way. Eventually, just let your attention flow with the enjoyable, rhythmic experience of the activity and let what comes come, i.e. zone out.

If you find you are getting distracted or caught up on a particular external thought, by all means come back to your breathing or another specific aspect of the activity before again letting your awareness expand. Don't try to experience a particular thought or feeling. As with meditation, the more you try to reach a higher level of experience, the less likely you are to do so. If your physiology is in a state conducive to a 'flow state' experience, you will naturally slip into it. If not, the experience will still be enjoyable and maximally effective for eliminating stress and connecting your mind and body. Either way, just enjoy it. As they say, *'just go with the flow'*!

Final note—exercise comfort, weight loss and stress management

Far from having transcendental experiences, in recent years exercise for many people has come to be seen as simply a means to lose weight or reduce stress. While exercise certainly has its place in regard to weight loss and stress management, these were traditionally seen to be supplementary to the higher purpose of creating greater mind-body connection. Many people reading this will question the idea of exercising according to ease and comfort as they equate vigorous exercise with being better for burning calories, losing weight or eliminating stress. However, it can be valuable to appreciate why this view is not necessarily ideal.

In our hectic, high-stress modern world, it can be easy to get out of balance. However, instead of reaping the true benefits of enjoyable exercise, many of us look to exercise, and more particularly high-intensity exercise, to address what is already out of balance—that is, to try to reduce stress and/or burn off calories that have resulted from excessive food consumption. Diagram 3 below illustrates a common cycle.

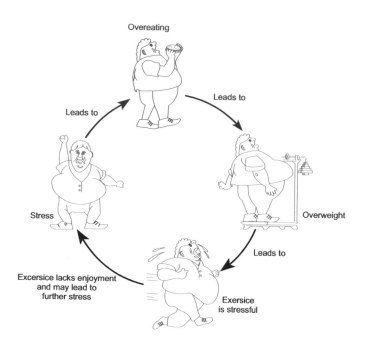

Diagram 3: Excessive stress commonly leads to overeating. Overeating leads to excess weight. Being overweight, and having a time-poor lifestyle, increases the tendency to over-exercise (i.e. exercise beyond what is comfortable) in order to burn off extra calories in the time available. This leads to exercise lacking enjoyment and even becoming a further stress in itself.

From a broader, natural wisdom perspective, the real problem here is not our inability to do enough strenuous exercise. If one enjoys regular, enjoyable exercise, in tune with the natural laws of health, but still has a problem with weight or stress, then something other than exercise is causing things to be out of balance. While it is not always easy, rather than trying to correct stress and/or overeating with exercise based on pushing beyond one's comfort zone ('I'm going to eat like a horse tonight, but I'll run it off tomorrow'), it is far healthier to address the underlying causes. This may involve starting a stress reduction technique, changing personal or work situations that are causing ongoing stress or simply learning to eat moderately in the first place. Diagram 4 illustrates how, by addressing the underlying stress, one will naturally tend to eat more healthily and maintain a more balanced weight, so can engage in exercise purely for its enjoyment.

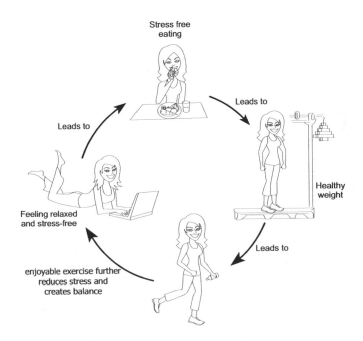

Diagram 4: Reducing stress leads to more balanced eating. More balanced eating leads to a healthier weight. A healthier weight allows one to exercise more from comfort and enjoyment rather than stress. Balanced, comfortable exercise further reduces stress.

Exercise is no doubt a great antidote to stress and an expanding waistline. Ideally, however, its highest purpose is not to compensate for other areas of our life being out of balance. By creating balance in life generally, like Mozart's music, exercise can be an unburdening, effortless and joyful experience—purely for the pleasure and fun of it. When we start to make pleasure and enjoyment the basis for being active, our motivation soars and we naturally want to exercise more.

Seed wisdom

In times past, exercise was seen as a means to reconnect to our deepest self and to experience the very core of who we are. Its purpose was not simply to lose weight, manage stress or have a firmer backside but to unite mind, body and spirit. In its highest form, exercise can be used as an active meditation to help culture higher levels of mind-body integration and open up the possibility of experiencing the ultimate paradox—moments of inner timelessness and transcendence within dynamic, outer activity.

The first step, however, is simply to reconnect to the intrinsic joy of movement. Exercise that is stressful or involves strain or pain ('no pain no gain') not only disconnects our mind and body, but also destroys Mother Nature's most fundamental source of motivation—enjoyment. When it comes to exercise, keep it simple. Just pick fun activities that involve moving your body. First and foremost do things you enjoy. Do what makes you dance.

Wisdom Five

Connect Daily with Mother Nature's Healing Gifts—earth, water, fire (sun), air and space

I go to nature to be soothed and healed,
and to have my senses put in order.
John Burroughs

Imagine our cosmic creator bestowed upon us five healing medicines and decreed that in order for us to enjoy good health, we simply needed to connect to them each day. The only catch was that these medicines would not be seen as medicines. They would be so basic and such an everyday part of life that we might very likely take them for granted. To a large degree, this is what has befallen us in many modernized parts of the world.

These medicines, or *'gifts from God'* as they have been known throughout time, come from the five fundamental elements that are known to comprise our universe: space, air, fire (sunshine), water and earth. The ancient cultures didn't just understand the five elements, but worshipped these gifts of nature as deities, gods or goddesses. In the Vedic tradition, the sun (Surya) is esteemed alongside famous Gods such as Brahma, Vishnu and Shiva. In other traditions there are Gods of air (Shu, Haya-Ji), water (Poseidon, Osiris) and of course Mother Earth herself (Gaia). All these gods or goddesses have been worshipped and given blessings in the hope that they would provide protection and nourishment in the areas of health for which they are responsible.

Ironically, at the same time as we are spending billions of dollars each year trying to detect genes responsible for cancer, we continue to create a cancerous world by poisoning the very environment we live in. We pollute our water, release harmful toxins into the air we breathe, poison our soils, add chemicals to our food, and overcrowd our cities. We live and work, more and more, in concrete jungles and high-rise buildings that are devoid of natural light, fresh clean air and visual beauty. Even our hospitals, where people supposedly go to get better, are generally cold, sterile, uninspiring places devoid of natural air, light and color. Such is our disconnection from Mother Nature's own medicinal pharmacy that we have even begun to see the sun's rays more as a source of danger than the wondrous health-promoting and healing gift that they are.

Is it any wonder we get sick?

Common to Okinawans, Vilcabambans, Abkhasians, Hunzans, Campodimelani and other healthy, long-living populations has been a close affinity to the natural world, and thus an intimate association with each of the five healing elements. While our modern world makes it challenging, there is much we can do individually to connect to our source elements. We will look at each in detail, starting with the one that is most misunderstood.

FIRE (SUNLIGHT)

The remover of all weakness, healer of all illness, Lord of all that stands and goes, He slays the demons and guards the worshippers.

A verse about the sun from the ancient Vedic text, *Rik Veda*.

It comprises the very center of our solar system. The life of our entire planet is dependent upon it. The food we eat is nothing but its stored energy. Literally and symbolically, it represents the eternal fire in nature and brings us light, color, energy, warmth and dynamism. It is the sun, and without it there could be no life. Unfortunately, today many people have almost come to think of the sun as evil because of its supposed links to skin cancer (more on that later), and have begun to distance themselves from this life-protecting jewel.

Despite a growing fear, the *sun is not out to KILL US!*

Ancient cultures of higher wisdom have known that healthy sun exposure is actually one of our greatest allies in our quest for health and happiness.

While too much sun is no doubt harmful, in the right amount at the right times (not when you may think), the sun does not cause skin cancer and in fact protects us from many cancers and much disease.

Why we need regular sun exposure

Our bodies need sunlight to manufacture the all-important vitamin D. Vitamin D plays a major role in all our vital bodily functions. These include gene expression, cell replication, calcium absorption and bone health, as well as the regulation of our immune system. Quite recent research has shown that immune system T cells do not become active without sufficient vitamin D. Direct sunlight exposure assists us in fighting infections, stimulates our brain chemistry, regulates our internal body clock, and even promotes balanced weight management through its effects on metabolic and thyroid functions.

In times past, and indeed up until just a few decades ago, most humans had significant direct exposure to sunlight each day. Today, with our busier 'indoor' lifestyles, many of us get up and go to work before the sun has much strength, work indoors all day, and come home when the sun is setting. Add in a growing fear of skin cancer, so even if people do go out in the sun, many cloak themselves in sun-shielding clothing or smother themselves in sunscreen. Apart from laborers and outdoor workers, the daily *direct* sunlight exposure for many people is often barely a few minutes. For those who work indoors and don't go outside for lunch, sometimes it is none at all. Despite an understandable education focus from authorities about the dangers of skin cancer, an unfortunate consequence is that many of us are now actually getting insufficient sun contact and are subjecting ourselves to significant vitamin D deficiency. Even in sun-drenched Australia, vitamin D deficiency is far more common than most people believe. Mild deficiency can affect up to 50% of the general population, particularly by the end of winter.[1] This can rise to 80% in at-risk populations such as veiled, dark-skinned pregnant women[2] and elderly or infirm residents who spend most of their time indoors.[3]

In the five years I've known about this problem and have recommended clients and friends get their vitamin D levels tested, less than a handful have come back with levels in the standard range, let alone the optimal range. Many people in the southern states of Australia, where there is less vitamin D producing UVB sun exposure, have had vitamin D levels less than one-quarter of the recommended levels.

The dangers of vitamin D deficiency

The overwhelming majority of research and research institutions around the world clearly associate vitamin D deficiency with a number of serious diseases. These include:

1. Osteoporosis—poor bone health[4]
2. Heart disease[5 8]
3. Depression—chronic fatigue / seasonal affective disorder[6 7]
4. Auto-immune disease such as rheumatoid arthritis[9], type 1 diabetes[5 8], ulcerative colitis[10] and multiple sclerosis[11 12]
5. <u>Cancers</u>: <u>breast</u>[13 14], <u>colon</u>[13 15 16], <u>prostate</u>[13 17 18], plus ten others[13]

In March 2002, one of the world's most prominent and respected vitamin D researchers, Dr William B. Grant, published studies linking the part of sunlight that helps us manufacture vitamin D (UVB) to cancer mortality rates in Caucasian Americans. Dr Grant showed inverse correlations for a total of fourteen different types of cancers. That is, as UVB sunlight exposure went down, the death rate from cancer went up. These cancers included many common ones such as breast, colon, non-Hodgkin's lymphoma and ovarian cancer. Other factors known to modify cancer risk, such as smoking or alcohol consumption, did not detract from this link.

From this and other research, it is estimated that anywhere between 20,000 and 60,000 cancer deaths annually in the US can be considered premature due to insufficient UVB sunlight exposure and vitamin D. A far higher number of people are diagnosed with cancer each year for the same reasons.[19]

While latitudinal variations between parts of the US and other countries would likely account for some differences in the extent of vitamin D deficiency, a similar risk to human health and even human life is undoubtedly occurring each year in other populations also.

A *sunny disposition*

Just as important as the physical benefits of sunlight are the sun's known effects of uplifting our mood and strengthening our emotional health. Modern research has shown for some time that vitamin D deficiency is associated with seasonal affective disorder (SAD). SAD relates to the depressive tendencies more prevalent in individuals living in low sunlight locations such as the United Kingdom. (Apparently, it's even more depressing than having to watch the English cricket team—though I would question if that's possible!) The visual effects of the sun are also critical for our emotional health. Sunlight is basically full-spectrum light in its most natural form. As such, it contains all the different wavelengths of light that are known to stimulate the different areas of our brain.

If we don't get sufficient natural light (sunlight) through our eyes, our brains cannot capture the required wavelengths of light to properly manufacture the neurotransmitters associated with joy and happiness.

This is why sunglasses should not be worn excessively. While they might be fashionable or 'look cool', they block the infusion of natural light into the brain. Over time, this can prevent the right balance of healthy brain chemistry being established.

Even before modern science confirms the full extent of the sun's benefits of stimulating our neurochemistry, we intuitively know that sunlight is good for us and lifts our spirits. When we think of 'feeling down' emotionally, we tend to correlate it with the qualities of heaviness, darkness and even the color black. It stands to reason that the sun, which is Mother Nature's most prominent and powerful source of light, brightness, energy and dynamism, should be a perfect antidote. Sunlight literally helps us create a more 'sunny' disposition and to counter feeling 'blue'. It 'lightens' our life and 'sparks' us up. If you come across people who are constantly feeling down or even depressed, and it's not a type of depression caused by life circumstances, consider if they may be 'malilluminated'. If so, a bit of healthy sun connection may be just the tonic they need.

Ancient sun wisdom—sun salutes, sun bathing and sun gazing

The ancients' view of the sun was quite different to our modern-day one. From the dawn of history, the sun has been worshipped by nearly every culture from the Iroquois and Plains peoples of North America to the ancient Persians and Babylonians. The ancient Egyptians worshipped the sun god Ra. In ancient Greece it was Apollo and Helios. As a means of healing, sun exposure has been used by the Aztecs, Incas, Mayans, Phonecians, Romans, Assyrians, Arabians, ancient Chinese, Japanese, Indians and many others. In former times, the sun's attributes were known to extend far beyond our current concept of vitamin D stimulation.

Three traditional practices highlight the natural wisdom connection between the sun and our mental, physical, emotional and spiritual health.

Surya Namaskar—the 'Salute to the Sun'

From ancient India to today, you have been able to go to the banks of the Ganges river each morning and see thousands of individuals performing the yoga practice of *'Surya Namaskar'* or Sun Salutations. While Surya Namaskar has recently become hugely popular in Western yoga centers for its wonderful physical strengthening and purifying effects, it was traditionally considered much more a spiritual than a physical practice.

In addition to its extraordinary benefits for mind and body, it is a practice designed to pay homage to the sun. It is literally a salutation or *'salute'* (Namaskar) to the sun (Surya). The sun was considered sacred and never taken for granted in ancient times. Such exercises were performed each morning to bless and give thanks to the sun for its light, warmth and energy, as well as to start each day imbibing these health and healing qualities into one's body.

Sun bathing

Sun bathing has been used to heal since the dawn of time. In contrast to our medical system dominated by pharmaceutical companies, Hippocrates, considered 'the Father of Medicine', rarely used drugs. He preferred natural medicines such as rest, water, air and gymnastic-type exercises. He was also a strong proponent of sunbathing and was known to practice it in the temple of Esculapius on one of the islands of ancient Greece.

Osteoporosis, or brittle bones, is a common ailment in the West these days. We hear a lot about the need for consuming sufficient calcium and performing weight-bearing exercise to strengthen our bones. What we don't hear so much about is that calcium absorption and thus the formation and maintenance of strong, healthy bones is substantially governed by vitamin D. Rarely is it mentioned that getting sufficient direct sunlight exposure is one of the most critical factors in ensuring optimal bone health. Many people who have osteoporosis and even bone cancer today are not even told to have their vitamin D status assessed. They are simply given calcium tablets or drugs. However, calcium in any form is largely useless without adequate levels of vitamin D. The calcium absorption and vitamin D link is analogous to a locked door and a key. Vitamin D is the key needed to unlock the door. Only if it unlocks the door can calcium move out of our intestines and enter our bloodstream.

In times past, in places such as India and Greece, if someone was suspected of weak bones, they weren't put on calcium supplements. In addition to being prescribed 'signature foods' that specifically nourish the bones, one of the first treatments was to 'sun bathe' for a short period each day. The same went for a number of other ailments, including circulatory problems, skin rashes and skin conditions such as psoriasis and eczema. In the right dose at the right time of day (in the middle of the day), sunlight was known to help nourish and heal the skin.

* It should be noted that sun bathing as mentioned here should not be confused with the modern-day practice of sunbaking for extended periods simply as recreation or to get a tan. The ancient practice of sun bathing was a deliberate act of sunning oneself for certain time periods, in order to deliver specific health benefits. The point is that deliberate, 'safe' sun exposure can heal.

Sun gazing

Another practice people were prescribed and engaged in during former times was known as 'sun gazing'. Sun gazing involves looking at the early morning or late setting sun. It was done within the first minutes of sunrise or last minutes of sunset, starting with just a few seconds and progressively increasing. Traditional Taoists and Shaolins have for centuries performed a similar practice called 'administering sunbeams'. They look toward rather than directly at the sun while doing various eye exercises.

Sun gazing was said to promote a number of psycho-spiritual and physical benefits. These include regulating the body clock, activating healthy immune and endocrine (hormone) function, increasing energy levels, reducing appetite, and improving eyesight and color perception. It may also be a powerful tonic to help address depressive tendencies caused by neuro-physiological deficiencies. This is due to the sun's direct effect of stimulating healthy brain chemistry. With the understanding that the energy we receive from eating food is basically just stored sunlight, it has been reported that some individuals have even survived for extended periods on nothing but water and imbibed sun energy through practices such as sun gazing.

The quality of the early morning sun is energizing and enlivening, while the setting sun is more calming and relaxing. Both inspire a powerful connection to Mother Nature and can bring profound spiritual benefits. Proponents of sun gazing say that if you extend one of your arms and place your open hand on the horizon, and the sun is below the top of your hand (i.e. below 10 degrees of arc), then the sun is safe to look at. They advise that just a few seconds is enough to begin with, increasing by a few seconds each day as long as the eyes are completely comfortable.

As far as I am aware, there is no mention in the traditional Ayurvedic texts to look at the sun with the eyes open. They do however state that indirect sunlight in the early morning is good for all individuals. Basically, if direct sun gazing is not for you, or you are in any doubt as to whether the sun is too high in the sky to be safe, err on the side of caution, and follow the Ayurvedic recommendation of looking at the sun with your eyes closed. This still confers many wonderful benefits without any risk to the eyes.

Skin cancer—don't make the sun the enemy

As the main reason you may be wary of exposing yourself to the sun is a fear of skin cancer or general sun damage, it can be good to consider a natural wisdom perspective on the issue. Right from the outset, I would like to say that I believe that the conventional advice to avoid sunning ourselves to such an extent that we burn our skin is undoubtedly good advice. Excessive sun exposure can not only damage our skin but also destroys vitamin D. It is certainly to be avoided. However, if sun exposure alone increases our risk of skin cancer, how do we account for the fact that:

1. ancient (and not so ancient) cultures who have spent far greater time in the sun without any protection—apart from their skin's own defenses—have generally survived rather well?

2. despite massive slip, slop, slap awareness campaigns and people avoiding the midday sun more and more, skin cancer rates are still at all-time highs?

3. the rates of malignant melanoma (the most harmful form of skin cancer) in fair-skinned *indoor workers* have been rising steadily and exponentially since 1940[20], while outdoor workers who often spend day after day in the sun, many without any protection, do not have an increasing rate of melanoma ... and many never get skin cancer?

4. according to Michael F. Holick, MD, PhD, one of the world's foremost experts on skin cancer, melanoma rarely occurs on the face and hands, the parts of the body that get the most direct sunlight exposure?[21]

At the very least, something does not seem to add up here. Even accepting arguments based on ozone depletion, differing skin pigmentation or problems of migration (the darker skin of most Native Americans for example is certainly more favorable to the harsh summer sun than fair-skinned individuals historically exposed to minimal sun), it seems odd that what was once known to be essential for every aspect of human health should suddenly be the sole cause of skin cancer.

Healthy (safe) sun exposure protects us from cancer and disease

When we are exposed to sunlight, our bodies produce substances such as melanin that protect our skin from UV radiation. Melanin is like our own natural sunscreen. When exposed to UVB sunlight, we also synthesize vitamin D, which, as discussed, is directly correlated with protection from many serious diseases including most common cancers.[a] Yet we are commonly advised to cover up or stay indoors during the middle of the day because it increases our risk of skin cancer, including melanoma. This is despite the fact that melanomas occur on parts

---

a   UV refers to general ultraviolet radiation from the sun. However, there are two main types of UV radiation that concern us—UVA and UVB. While both UVA and UVB can damage the skin, excessive UVA is more closely linked to increased melanoma risk as it penetrates deeper into the skin. Importantly, only UVB radiation produces vitamin D.

of the body that get the least amount of regular sun exposure. Even if this anomaly was due to melanomas spreading, illness tends to manifest in the weakest part of the body—the 'weakest link in the chain' analogy. Why are the least exposed areas the weakest link?

The most likely reason is that the sun, in repeated small and safe doses, actually protects us from cancer.

If you go to the gym once every three months, your muscles will likely get sore and ache the next day, as they are not prepared for what you're exposing them to. If, however, you expose your muscles to moderate weight training on most days of the week, they will adapt accordingly. They will tolerate more and more weight without any adverse side effects. It is the same with sun exposure. Our skin cells, like all our other body cells, have an innate intelligence, and when they are exposed to moderate sunlight regularly over time, they adapt by building up the appropriate pigmentation and biochemical defenses. Other areas of our body also begin sending the necessary resources to the skin to deal with any increased sunlight exposure. Additionally, when we get regular exposure to UVB sunlight, we optimize our vitamin D level, which further assists our bodies to resist illness over time. With adequate vitamin D and appropriate skin defenses, even if we were to get *too much sun* on a particular day, our bodies will generally have the ability to counteract any damage before it becomes hazardous.

The reality is that small, safe, regular exposures of sunlight provide us with far more protection than does wrapping ourselves up in cotton wool for weeks on end and then going out on a weekend and spending hours in the sun. This is of course what many of us do, particularly office workers. Research shows that people who work indoors and then go out in the sun on weekends are one of the highest risk groups for skin cancer. We are more likely to get sunburnt this way and this has been linked to increased melanoma rates.[22] Such a sporadic method of sun exposure subjects our skin cells to more damage and a greater propensity to replicate (become pre-cancerous or cancerous) due to a reduced vitamin D level. According to a 2009 study abstract from the US Food and Drug Administration's Center for Devices and Radiological Health, indoor workers get three to nine times 'less' solar UV exposure than outdoor workers, yet have an increasing incidence of melanoma, whereas outdoor workers do not.[23] Let's repeat that. Those who stay indoors for large parts of the day and get significantly less UV exposure have an '*increasing*' risk of melanoma. It is hypothesized that the reason for this is that indoor workers have low levels of vitamin D in their skin—due to low UVB sunlight exposure—as well as having increased UVA exposure. UVA can pass through windows and break down vitamin D.

> Avoiding the sun, staying indoors (e.g. working all day indoors) or blocking all sunlight exposure by always 'covering up' is certainly no way to avoid skin cancer or to ensure optimal health.
>
> While fairer-skinned individuals need to be careful to avoid 'overexposure', never distance yourself from the sun so much that you can't accept its gifts of brightness, power, energy, dynamism, emotional wellbeing and physical health.

Connecting to the sun—Ideas to help

1. Welcome and gives thanks to the sun each morning.

Sun permitting, go outside and spend a few minutes in the early morning sun. Give thanks for the sun and welcome its gifts of warmth, light and healing into your life.

2. Get your vitamin D level assessed.

If you haven't done so recently, get a blood test to assess your vitamin D level ('serum 25 OH' or 'hydroxyvitamin D3'). This is the first step to determining your vitamin D health and could literally save your life.

3. Let the sun heal you.

Skin Conditions: If you have a cut, rash, skin infection or even a condition such as eczema or psoriasis, try some 'middle of the day' summer sun exposure on the site for a few minutes each day. Spending time in the ocean or having salt water baths can also be of benefit for such conditions.

Eye Health: To improve your general eye health, get some indirect early morning sunlight through your eyes whenever you can, and at anytime of the day look towards the sun with your eyes 'closed'. Lightly massage the eyelids and around your eyes at the same time to help stimulate your color perception.

Mood lifter/Emotion balancer: If you are feeling a little down, heavy or negative, where conditions allow it, be sure to get adequate sun exposure, both in the early morning and during the middle of the day. Even if there is no sunlight as such in the early morning, being exposed to the natural UV light will still be helpful.

4. Get regular, small (safe) sunlight exposure whenever possible

i) Use the 'shadow rule'

In order to get sun exposure for optimal vitamin D synthesis, use the shadow rule. When your shadow is 'shorter' than you are, expose as much skin as you can for an appropriate time period (see ii. below). For most parts of Australia, these times will be during the midday hours—10am to 2pm—in the warmer months of the year. If you work indoors, be sure to get outside at lunchtime for some direct sun exposure.

ii) Get an appropriate level of exposure for 'you'

The exact duration for optimal (safe) vitamin D sun exposure depends on factors such as the strength of the sun, your age and skin type—the darker your skin, the more sun exposure you require. As a general guide, 'expose your hands, face and arms to one-third of the amount that produces a faint redness of your skin most days.'[24] If you are vitamin D deficient, look to 'expose as much of your skin as possible (don't scare the neighbors) to the point just before the faintest pink coloring'. That is, if you 'pinken' in 30 minutes, expose yourself for approximately 20—25 minutes each side of your body. If you 'pinken' in 10 minutes, sun for 7 minutes each side.[25]

5. For more information on

- why you need to get your vitamin D sun exposure in the 'middle' of the day
- how factors such as nutrition and the use of sunscreens and commercial soaps can affect skin health, and thus the possibility of skin cancer
- current recommendations regarding optimal vitamin D levels
- ways to improve your vitamin D status should you be deficient

read the full sun connection article at www.markbunn.com.au/Sunlight_AvoidItAtYourPeril

* A more detailed 'Ideas to help' section also appears in the supplementary ebook.

EARTH

Earth, thou great footstool of our God, who reigns on high; thou fruitful source of all our raiment, life, and food; our house, our parent, and our nurse.

Isaac Watts

The most fundamental of Mother Nature's gifts is her very own body, the physical earth.

The need for us to 'earth' ourselves on a regular basis has been lost over the last few decades, especially in our modern cities. Without close contact with the earth, we can become more susceptible to a number of mental and physical imbalances. Conditions such as anxiety, mood swings, irrational behavior, insomnia, restlessness, and digestive and elimination disorders can all be aggravated by distancing ourselves from our physical foundation. The ancients knew that we humans were intimately connected to the land. Far from being an inert, unchanging mass of rock, the earth was seen by cultures as diverse as the Mayans, American Indians and African pygmies as a living, breathing, pulsating organism within itself. The Australian Aboriginal Dreamtime stories also reflect this.

By its very nature, the earth provides stability, support and nourishment. We call the earth '*the ground*' and when we lose connection with the physical foundation of our planet, we can lose that intangible stability and support in our own lives. We become unsettled, spacey or 'ungrounded'. Think of our world over the last few decades. We spend a part of our lives thousands of meters in the air flying from one part of the world to another. We land on concrete, get shuttled across town in a car, bus or train to a two- or three-storey house or a high-rise building. Some of us then work all day in 50-storey skyscrapers. Weeks can go by with us barely setting foot on a living, breathing patch of soil. This is standard practice for inner-city living around the world. Is it any wonder that sleep problems, anxiety, stress, feeling lost, spacey or un-grounded are starting to be seen in epidemic proportions?

As humans, we are designed to live in harmony with planet Earth. This literally means 'living with' the earth. It means being physically connected to the soil, the trees and the grass. Most Native American cultures understood that just as our bodies have their own unique vibrational energy, so too does the earth itself. When we spend time connected to the earth, it is as if we recalibrate our own energy field with the universal energy field of nature. This rebalances, harmonizes and strengthens our body's vibrational resonance. We maintain the vibration of physical vitality and stay mentally grounded and 'in tune' with the world around us.

Cherokee Indian tradition suggests that there is an energy that sits just above the ground—about 60cm high. This energy field is known to have its own particular vibration and nourishing effect when we are in contact with it. The reason tassles are often worn in many traditional cultures is that they are thought to help circulate this energy around the body. The limited clothing common to Aboriginal cultures is also in part due to their understanding that excessive clothing can obstruct one's connection to this energy field. If you have ever seen an individual or group doing tai chi, you may have noticed a pose where they bend down towards the ground and make a scooping up motion with their hand. In its essence, this action is literally about scooping up energy from this field to bring it into the body.

Mia Dalby-Ball is an Australian woman who has spent much time learning from indigenous elders. A Cherokee teacher of hers explained that children today can often spend much of their time above the earth's energy field due to being in prams, high cots or spending long periods indoors. She recommended that one of the best things for young children, especially if they are upset or don't seem 'their usual self' is to let them spend some time crawling or playing at ground level.

Happy campers—happy gardeners

Keep close to Nature's heart ... and break clear away, once in a while, and climb a mountain or spend a week in the woods. Wash your spirit clean.

John Muir

Another common feature of many traditional cultures is that if someone *'loses their way'* in life, they are not sent off to a psychiatrist or told to get a prescription. Instead, the wise elders or tribal healers will often recommend that they pack up a little knapsack, take a few days' supplies and head out to the bush. This is often done along with a designated elder guide. Just this process of getting back to the land can often completely re-orientate a person's life. They get the space to clear their mind. The clean bush air and bright sunshine enliven their spirit. Bathing in streams of fresh, running water cleanses their body and soul. Sleeping on the earth, they reconnect and ground themselves with Mother Nature's nurturing bosom. Campers and those that spend time in nature often report equally transformative experiences. Maybe that's where the expression 'happy campers' comes from. Such practices should still be recommended today. Mother Nature is a wonderful healer.

Many years ago I had a client named Judy. Judy was in her mid-40s and had been diagnosed with early stages of osteoporosis (brittle bones). She was advised to increase her exercise levels, particularly some resist-ance-type weight training. She assumed that meant going to the gym. I asked Judy if she liked going to the gym. The gloomy look on her face said it all, but she added, 'I can't think of anything worse than going to a place full of muscle-bound grunting, sweaty guys and lycra-laden women while doing exercises I can't stand in a room reeking of B.O.' I took that as a no. I then asked her if she liked gardening. Well, now her face could have lit up a concert hall. 'Oh, I love gardening. My garden is my sanctuary. Unfortunately, I've been so busy the last few years that it has become a bit neglected.' I said, 'Judy, why don't you spend the time you currently do at the gym, working in your garden?' She replied as I had expected. 'Well, I'd love to, but now with my bones and all, it's really a priority that I go to the gym to get my exercise. My health is more important than my garden.' With a half-sympathetic and a half-excited smile, I replied, 'Do you really think your leg muscles know the difference between doing leg lunges with a 10 kg barbell at the gym and squatting down in your garden to lift up a 10 kg rock? Do you think your shoulders, arms and abdominal muscles know the difference between doing bicep curls in the gym (while having to look at some guy admiring his own biceps) and pulling out tough weeds or lifting a wheelbarrow full of soil? Do you think your heart and lungs know the difference between you stepping on the step machine and walking, squatting, lunging and stepping around your garden?'

After getting my point, Judy replied, 'Well no, apart from the time I would save not having to drive through the traffic to get to the gym, the air would be a hell of a lot cleaner and I would actually enjoy gardening so I would probably do it for longer, and my muscles, joints and bones would probably end up getting a lot more benefits.' Although I, like many people, enjoy going to gyms, I couldn't have said it any better myself.

Enjoying the many benefits of our modern way of living is wonderful, but to also enjoy our best health, we need to regularly ground ourselves by connecting with the earth.

Indoor Earthing Products

Recent studies have begun showing how regularly 'earthing' ourselves can promote natural self-healing mechanisms and potentially reduce many modern-day health conditions and chronic illnesses. New, 'indoor' earthing products have also been developed to enable us to get the same benefits of earthing, while living and working indoors.

For more information, see www.markbunn.com.au/earthing &/or www.earthinginstitute.net

---

Connecting to the earth—Ideas to help

1. At every opportunity, sit down on the grass, get out in the garden or walk in a park. If you live or work in a high-rise building or apartment, be extra vigilant about grounding yourself in these ways.

2. Where practical, take your shoes and socks off and walk on the ground with bare feet. If you do yoga, tai chi or other similar exercises in the mornings, where appropriate do them barefoot on the ground.

3. If you suffer from poor sleep, anxiety or anything related to feeling excessively 'spacey', consider if there may be any correlation with beginning to live or work in a high-rise building, especially an inner-city one, or becoming ungrounded in some way.

4. Get out of town and back to nature every now and then. Visit a national park or 'go bush' for an occasional holiday. It doesn't have to be 'pitch a tent' type camping, just anywhere that gets you back to the grounding energy of Mother Earth.

WATER

Water, then, is the most beautiful element ... rich in usefulness ... purifies from all filth, and not only from the filth of the body but from that of the soul ...

John of Damascus

Literally and symbolically, water has been seen as a 'gift from heaven'. This is very different to our modern age, when we barely give water a second thought, until we so pollute our waterways or waste what we have that we hardly have any fresh water left. In ancient cultures throughout Europe, Asia and the Middle East, water was seen as a natural medicine. As in modern-day hydrotherapy, the ancients honored water for its purifying, cleansing and revitalizing properties, particularly within the body.

Having sufficient water in our cells is critical for us to absorb and transport nutrients. It is imperative for us to effectively flush out toxins and eliminate wastes, and the estimated ten billion biochemical reactions that take place in our cells each second are completely dependent on it. Think of a garden in the middle of a drought. Without water, everything dies. It's the same with our bodies. When in a healthy state, our bodies are over 70% water, so we need to water them regularly. Although it's not rocket science, due to our busy lives, eating insufficient fruits and vegetables (which naturally have a high water content) and regularly consuming alcohol and caffeine drinks (both of which dehydrate the body), many of us live in a perpetual state of internal drought. Every day we compromise our health simply by not drinking enough water. The greatest problem is that most people don't appreciate the huge problems that such a simple disconnection from the major constituent of our body brings us. Let's have a look at just a few examples.

Headaches

Our brains consist of over 80% water when in their optimally hydrated state. If we get dehydrated, our brain does too. A dehydrated brain not only functions less effectively but it also shrinks. Eventually it can shrink to the point of causing pain. That pain, along with our thirst mechanism—which we are often too busy to tune into—is our body's way of letting us know that it doesn't have enough water to function properly. Instead of simply drinking more water, we commonly pop a headache pill or pain killer. The pain, which is just a symptom, is killed off, but we remain dehydrated and the problem remains unaddressed. Dehydration is obviously not the only cause of headaches. It is, however, a common one, and can often be corrected without popping pills, by drinking a couple of glasses of warm water and maintaining good hydration.

Fatigue

Eating good quality, high-intelligence food can still result in low energy levels if we fail to consume enough water. Even the best nutrition in the world can't get where it is needed if there is insufficient water in our cells to effectively transport it there. Water provides the optimal environment for the efficient transportation of nutrients, and catalyses the metabolic reactions that produce our energy.

Water is not just cleansing, it is energizing.

Many people live each day 'not quite feeling 100%' in terms of their energy and vitality. While they often put it down to age, diet or lack of sleep and possibly spend hundreds of dollars on energy supplements, an all too common cause is sub-optimal hydration. If you are low on energy, get constantly tired or have some form of ongoing fatigue, check your connection to the element of water, meaning how much of it you are drinking.

High blood pressure

Insufficient water in our body can stagnate our blood. This restricts blood flow and constricts the circulatory channels. In such situations, the pressure on our blood vessels needs to increase in order to get sufficient blood to our tissues. Allowed to occur regularly, this can lead to high blood pressure.

Constipation

Fiber tablets or fiber supplements are often the first thing people think of to relieve constipation. They can sometimes help, but it's not always because of the fiber. Many times, it's the fact that the tablet or supplement has been taken with a glass of 'water'! Dehydration, or lack of water, is often the problem. Without water, things 'dry up', including our bowels. That's why real foods, Mother Nature's fruits, vegetables and cooked wholegrains, are the best medicine of all. Together they are packed with fiber in its natural form and have a naturally high water content. One of the first steps for alleviating constipation is to reduce mental stress, eat high water content whole foods and drink plenty of warm water. Water helps lubricate the stools and warm water helps 'soften the pipes'—much like warming a garden hose makes it softer and more pliable. This enables the waste matter to move out more freely.

Obesity

Having insufficient water in the body compromises the effective elimination of metabolic by-products from our cells. This not only leads to the accumulation of wastes within the body, but also disrupts proper cellular functioning. This in turn can upset our sense of food satiety, disturb proper food cravings and create unbalanced energy levels. When our energy levels are low and our natural cravings are disturbed, eating beyond our body's needs is far more likely. For many people who regularly overeat, it's not more food they need but more water. Staying optimally hydrated not only improves the elimination of wastes, it reduces the likelihood of over-indulging and is thus one of the best ways to maintain a healthy weight. To eat less and weigh less ... drink more!

DNA repair and serious disease

Sufficient water flow throughout the body is needed for all cellular functioning and repair. If we restrict our water intake, not only do we impair our body's general performance, we can affect our DNA's ability to heal itself. Our DNA is constantly under threat by free radicals and other invaders, which can jeopardize its intelligent functioning if it cannot properly protect itself. It needs sufficient water to do this. Lack of water in the body generally will compromise the ability of DNA to repair itself, to oversee the repair of damaged cells, and to correct breakdowns in cellular memory. The more this occurs over time, the greater the like-lihood of impaired functioning and thus imbalance and disease.

Many people live in a permanent state of dehydration. They then spend thousands of dollars on pharmaceutical pills, potions, home co-lonics and visits to health farms to remedy their headaches, constant fatigue, constipation, high blood pressure and many other conditions. However, just by drinking enough water each day and refraining from overloading their digestive systems with too much processed food, their bodies could more easily flush out toxins, self-cleanse and self-purify. Additionally, by drinking less coffee, alcohol and softdrinks, some peo-ple could even correct a number of serious health conditions over time.

Connect to water externally as well

The ancients understood that our connection to the element of wa-ter is not just in terms of the water we take internally. They knew that in addition to being energizing and cleansing, water by nature is cooling, lubricating and soothing. Connection to the element of water helps calm and relax our nervous system. Research has shown how things like hav-ing a fish tank or listening to running water can reduce our blood pres-sure and normalize our heart beat. In our fast-paced, mentally stimulat-ing world, a close connection to the element of water can be extremely beneficial in helping us maintain both physiological and psychic balance. Natural bodies of water such as the ocean not only provide visual beauty, the actual water itself cleanses the spirit, enlivens the senses and helps nourish mind, body and emotions. Most of us know the relaxing effects of sitting by a lake, the energizing effects of walking along a pristine beach, and the exhilaration of diving into Mother Nature's swimming pool—the ocean. It may be no coincidence that the massive sea change movement of the last couple of decades has coincided with the corresponding surge in modern-day technology and nervous system stimulation.

While we can't all live near the ocean, fish tanks, water features or small fountains or ponds in a garden can all help nourish and balance the feeling level of a home or office. Even pictures of seascapes, waterfalls and lakes, or playing music with the sound of flowing rivers, falling rain or waves crashing, can produce profoundly calming effects and soothe the emotions.

Connecting to water—Ideas to help

1. If you suffer from headaches, ongoing fatigue, listlessness, poor concentration, constipation, lightheadedness, high blood pressure, obesity or problems related to excessive heat (e.g. anger, ulcers, burning of any kind), ask yourself, 'How is my connection to the element of water?', 'Am I drinking enough water?'

2. Do not blindly drink eight glasses or two liters of water a day as is commonly recommended. (See the ebook for more on why this is often far less than ideal). To know how much water a day you should drink, stop regularly to tune in to your body's inner wisdom regarding thirst and regularly check the color of your urine. It should be clear or light yellow.

3. Drink 'moving' water. When water flows, it breaks down into its component parts: hydrogen and oxygen. This releases energy. It is the 'flow' of water that energizes it and helps it penetrate into the cells of our body to do its cleansing and purifying work. In the absence of a natural stream flowing through your living room, refill water cups from a water dispenser or from filtered tap water. If using a water bottle or thermos that has been sitting stationary for an hour or two, gently tip it back and forth a few times before drinking from it.

4. If you don't live near a large body of water, or if you work in an environment that has a dry or busy quality to it, look to introduce a small aspect of the water element into that space, e.g. a fish tank or water feature.

5. Appreciate that water is life and therefore you can transform your life by strengthening your connection to this life-giving element.

AIR

I know that our bodies were made to thrive only in pure air, and the scenes in which pure air is found.

John Muir

Have you ever been in a modern apartment or housing complex where the building next door was so close that there was almost no movement of air? Have you worked in an office building that only had artificial ventilation? When you drive out into the country, is the first thing that hits you just how fresh and clean the air is? Do you stop and take a few deep breaths because it is so revitalizing? Arguably the most intimate of all things related to life itself is the air we breathe. Yet, just like the food we eat, the quality of the air we take in can either exhilarate and enliven us, just barely allow us to survive or, worse still, promote sickness and disease.

While we generally think of oxygen as the key component in the air we breathe, traditional healers understood that it is the prana or lifeforce content of air that is most important. Whether the air we breathe dulls or enlivens us, i.e. gives us life, is dependent on how much life-force it has rather than merely its oxygen content. It is the life-force or life energy that is most critical in all of Mother Nature's gifts—air, water, soil, food—and the ancients knew that it is most lively when these elements are in their purest, most unadulterated state. Just as old, stale, highly processed food is devoid of life-force, so is old, stagnant, polluted air. Like water, air also needs to move in order to maintain its life-force and energize us. Electricity is the movement, or *flow*, of electrons. If there is no flow, there is no electricity or power. Similarly, flowing or circulating air has a charge of energy. It is this charge that 'recharges' us. That's why outside air, assuming it's clean, is more invigorating than indoor air. If we spend a day in a poorly ventilated building or live in a smoggy city, by the end of the day we might still be living but it is doubtful whether we will feel truly 'alive'. In contrast, spending time near a fresh ocean breeze or in a pristine rainforest invigorates our entire mind, body and spirit. Such air is Mother Nature's breath of life.

Bring nature to you

For anyone living in or near a modern industrialized city, breathing fresh, pure air is simply not possible. While air purifiers and humidifiers may provide some benefits, one of the best ways to naturally improve the quality of air we breathe is to bring Mother Nature to us. If the wind is Mother Nature's breath, the plant kingdom is her lungs. Plants take in our waste gases (carbon dioxide) and in return give us fresh oxygen and life-force. They also absorb pollutants and other toxins from the air, making it cleaner and healthier.

A number of studies, including those headed by Professor Margaret Burchett of the University of Technology, Sydney, have found that pot plants can reduce air toxins such as carbon dioxide by 10-25% and carbon monoxide by up to 90%.[26] Burchett's team has also demonstrated how various plants can reduce total volatile organic compounds or VOC's by up to 75%.[27] VOC's are chemical compounds often found in high levels in modern buildings due to outgassing from plastic or synthetic materials such as new paint, synthetic carpets and modern furnishings. VOC's are not good for our health. Other studies have shown reduced absenteeism in schoolchildren who have plants in their classroom, and that potted plants in workplaces can reduce sick leave by up to 60%.[28]

Even more than simply cleaning our air, the ancients understood that plants are cooling by nature and provide a balancing 'lunar' energy. As night is to day, a plant's lunar or moon energy makes it a perfect antidote to the hot, solar energy of computers and mobile phones.

Connecting to air—Ideas to help

1. If you are exercising and it is practical to do so, walk, jog or ride in natural settings, e.g. near trees, parks or gardens rather than main roads, concrete jungles or indoors.
2. Have at least one green plant in each main room of your house, in your office and near your computer. Palms, ferns and spider plants are good choices as they are excellent for air purification as well as being visually pleasing and low maintenance.
3. When going away, occasionally give polluted cities a miss. Go bush or to a country location where you can get some natural, clean air.
4. Where practical, allow the air in your home or workplace to circulate. Open doors and windows where appropriate or use ceiling or portable fans if needed.
5. If you feel that you sleep well but you still wake up less than fully revitalized, check that you have fresh, circulating air in your bedroom.

SPACE

In minds crammed with thoughts, organs clogged with toxins and bodies stiffened with neglect, there is just no space for anything else.

Alison Rose Levy

From the understanding of Ayurveda, in addition to the elements of earth, water, fire and air, space is considered a fundamental element. Although we don't usually think of space as an element in itself, without space none of the other elements could exist. Scientists tell us that our world is in essence 99.999% empty space (in reality, this space is far from empty), yet we don't always consider the effect space has on our health. Indigenous cultures have understood that how we think and feel is significantly affected by the space around us. Space-clearing ceremonies have been performed as an integral part of life by the elders, or shamans, from the Celtics, Tibetan Buddhists and many Native American tribes. To them, clearing and cleansing the spaces that we inhabit is critical in order that the all-important life energy can flow unimpeded. Being intimately connected to their physical environment, they also knew that clearing the space about them could release many of the negative physical and emotional attachments they had to the space.

Our experience usually confirms that when we have adequate space around us, we are better able to think in more expansive, broad-ranging ways. Home magazines and real estate advertisements commonly feature large, open living areas looking out over expansive, panoramic views of natural settings: trees, water, nature. This is because such views create pleasure, expansion, balance and a lack of limitation in the way we think and feel. Chefs, artists and designers who have only tiny spaces to work in often complain that this stifles their creativity. Our brains and the neural pathways associated with spatial organization are constantly taking in information from our environment. When we are physically cramped or our living space is full of 'junk', we can feel on a subtle, subconscious level that our thinking is adversely affected. When our bodily channels become blocked, we become physically sick. When our personal space gets blocked or cluttered, we can become psychically sick.

> In Ayurveda, it is clearly stated that we don't just metabolize what we eat, we metabolize everything that we experience through our senses.
>
> Mess, congestion or clutter in our outer environment is likely to result in congested or cluttered thinking in our inner environment.

> ### Connecting to space—Ideas to help
>
> 1. Consider your living and/or working environment. If it feels heavy rather than light, or blocked and congested rather than clear and open, look to declutter the physical space around you. Minimize the junk and create order in your immediate environment whenever you can.
> 2. If you regularly struggle with mental overload, cloudy thinking or lack of clarity in your decision-making, throw out all the things you never use anymore. If any clothes, furnishings or personal belongings give you a sense of heaviness or simply don't energize and inspire you, give them away.

Seed wisdom

Health has become so complicated and scientific that we can lose sight of the fact that the most powerful medicines for a vibrant, happy life exist right under our noses. They are available to us in abundance every day and are completely free of charge. Common to populations with high numbers of long-living, healthy individuals has been daily access to adequate space, fresh air, direct sunlight, clean water and a close contact with the earth. Before worrying about the latest health fads and gimmicky wellness products, don't lose sight of the simple wisdoms and everyday pillars of Mother Nature's eternal health recipe. Connect with the earth, drink plenty of water, get regular sunlight exposure (in moderation), breathe in fresh, clean air wherever possible and ensure sufficient space in your life. Never forget ... the simplest things are always the best.

Wisdom Six

Enliven Inner Silence

*It is only when we silent the blaring sounds of our daily existence
that we can finally hear the whispers of truth that life reveals to
us, as it stands knocking on the doorsteps of our hearts.*

K.T. Jong

Imagine a beautiful fruit tree is growing in your garden, and it is your job to ensure its optimal health. If you didn't understand that the true source of the tree (its roots) lies underground, you might spend many hours watering all the external parts of the tree individually—the trunk, branches, leaves and fruits. If you did this, the tree would soon die because you didn't nourish its source. However, although the roots of a tree lie underground and cannot be seen with the naked eye, you know that they are the ultimate source of nourishment for the entire tree. By spending a few minutes each day watering the roots, i.e. tending to what lies 'unseen', you would nourish every part of the tree and enjoy bountiful fruit for many years. This analogy comes from Maharishi Mahesh Yogi, the renowned Indian scholar and spiritual teacher. According to Maharishi, the exact same idea applies to our success in life. He says,

'Water the roots to enjoy the fruits.' In other words, to have balanced health and success in life (enjoy the fruits), we need to nourish our unseen, non-physical, spiritual source (water our roots).

Wise teachers from Jesus to Buddha, Krishna to Mohammed, Shaolin monks to Aboriginal elders, Hippocrates to Einstein, have also known that the unseen or spiritual part of us is the essential nourishing source of all that we are. Throughout time, there has always been one consistent message amongst all the great philosophies and spiritual precepts. That is, due to the ever-changing nature of our material world, permanent happiness can never be attained by tending to the physical level of life alone. We can race around day after day, year after year, focusing on the external areas of our lives—diet, exercise, work, relationships—yet, despite much effort, happiness can still elude us. The secret of true fulfillment, we have been told, lies within. Jesus said, 'The kingdom of heaven is within.' The underlying message of the Tao Te Ching is that 'The Tao (the eternal source of all that exists) is within you.' Perhaps Socrates summed it up most succinctly with his famous words, 'Know Thyself.'

Despite this age-old wisdom, in today's world of instant gratification, on-demand information and entertainment saturation, how many of us stop to nourish our silent source within? We wake up to alarm clocks ringing in our ears. We shower while listening to radio DJ's belting out the day's breaking news. We get dressed in front of the TV, read the paper while eating breakfast, make phone calls while driving to work. When we go for a walk or run, we don't leave without taking our iPod. While 'silence is golden' for some, the thought of spending a minute alone or in quiet contemplation is for many a scary thought. We have created such a God of activity in our Western world that we have largely forgotten one of the most fundamental tenets of life—that inseparable from all intelligent, evolutionary activity is 'non-activity.' Everything in our universe is built on the cycles of activity and rest, rest and activity. We have day and then night, summer then winter, inhalation then exhalation, heart pump then heart relax. Claude Debussy once said, 'Music is the *space* between the notes'. Just as it is in the spaces that music gets created, the ancients tell us that it is only in the spaces between our thoughts that we can truly enjoy the 'music in our lives'.

> It is in the silence between our thoughts that we access our highest creativity, our deepest intuitions and our most profound joys. When our minds become so crammed with 'noise', we block the subtle, divine impulses that are there to guide us to our highest health.
>
> As the Tao beautifully declares, 'You remain silent and it speaks, you speak and it remains silent'.

Recent discoveries in modern science have begun to confirm the wisdom of our ancestors. In the past two decades, quantum physics has discovered that underlying our minds and bodies is a non-physical field of energy and intelligence. This field, from which all the energy and matter of our material world are said to emanate, exists at the basis of our entire universe. It underlies everything from our subtlest thoughts and the beating of our hearts to the movement of the planets. When science describes this non-localized field, it correlates precisely with that of traditional cultures and the age-old natural sciences when describing the spiritual realm of life. Science calls it the 'unified field'. The ancient Vedas refer to it as a 'field of consciousness'. Thousands of Native American tribes may be referring to the very same thing when they talk about the 'spirit that moves through all things'. Other traditions refer to 'source', 'universal intelligence' and even 'God'. Regardless of its name, both modern science and ancient wisdom, East and West, point to the same fundamental realization. At the basis of all that we are is an infinite reservoir of energy, dynamism, creativity, intelligence and power. Most importantly, like a limitless treasure trove, the yogic masters have declared that if we simply know how to contact and enliven this inner field of life, we can begin to command more of this energy, creativity and intelligence in our own lives. The eternal question is: how do we do this?

Transcending—nourishing the silent source of all

When we transcend our capacities, immediately we get an inner joy, an inner thrill, which is another name for perfection. No perfection can ever be achieved without self-transcendence.

Sri Chinmoy

When I was nineteen, my darling sister and wise brother-in-law, a state cricketer at the time, had just been taught the Transcendental Meditation (or TM) technique. They mentioned that their teacher had taught a lot of highly successful athletes and business people and suggested that I might also like to learn as a way to help my football career— they obviously thought that I needed all the help I could get! Within days, I was sitting in a corporate office in the heart of Melbourne's business district, about to learn the ancient mental art of transcending.

My instruction began by watching a videotape of Maharishi, the man who brought TM to the West. Maharishi was a small yet strongly built man with a long, full beard. He sat cross-legged in a white robe and waved a bright yellow rose as he explained his famous analogy of 'watering the root to enjoy the fruit'. To a teenage Western 'jock' footballer, all this was certainly a new experience to say the least! However, as he illuminated some of the most profound wisdoms of life while laughing and giggling like a small child, he seemed to be the happiest person I'd ever seen. I was on the edge of my seat, wanting to learn his secret.

Maharishi went on to discuss how the human mind is just like an ocean. On the surface of the ocean, many waves come and go, rising up and crashing down. This is like the many thoughts that continually rise up in our busy minds. However, at the bottom of an ocean, everything is perfectly calm and silent. Likewise, at the deepest level of who we are is a silent, infinitely calm ocean of 'consciousness.' It was suggested that by connecting to this inner field of consciousness we become like a boat dropping an anchor to the depths of the ocean floor. Regardless of how rough the waves on the surface of the ocean may be, if the boat is securely anchored, it can ride out any storm. Similarly, if we anchor ourselves to our inner, unbounded spiritual source, the inevitable ups and downs of life, which are the nature of the material world, gradually fail to disturb us so much. To use another analogy, like being in the eye of a hurricane we are better able to remain relaxed, calm and silent within, despite the noisy winds of life blowing all around us. What really got my attention, however, was when Maharishi detailed how this unbounded, inner field was not at all difficult to contact. In fact, he explained that the common belief that meditation or spiritual growth requires much discipline and effort was indeed a complete misunderstanding. It was pointed out that the experience of happiness is in reality completely natural for our mind, and with the right mental training each of us can access this silent, inner field in the most effortless way. Though this all sounded wonderful, I had had enough of the theory and wanted to experience this inner field of consciousness for myself. Soon enough my wish was granted. I was taught the timeless art of transcending and within minutes I had an experience I will never forget.

Having been given a mantra, a sound that promotes transcending, and specific instruction in how to use it, I began to meditate. Like it was only yesterday, I remember almost instantaneously falling into a deep state of pure relaxation. It was like I was sinking down within myself. Soon my body became completely still. My breathing slowed almost to a state of suspension and the endless chatter of my mind, which was usually my constant companion, seemed to evaporate away. I was not asleep, and in fact was more awake than I had ever been. I continued to sink deeper and deeper into a state of profound peace, while my mind seemed to be expanding and expanding. I was so completely relaxed that I could not feel the boundaries of my physical body, yet I was completely alert. It was like I was silently observing the whole process and I felt that I had temporarily glimpsed what the yogis of times past meant by the term '*witnessing*'.

After floating in what felt like a private sea of happiness for about twenty minutes, I was brought back to my usual, comparatively mundane level of experience by the voice of the teacher. I was informed that what I had temporarily experienced was what Maharishi called the state of '*restful alertness*.' The body experiences deep relaxation while the mind is perfectly clear and awake. It was explained that when one dips a white cloth into colored dye, each time the cloth is taken out it retains a little more of the color. Similarly, after dipping into the silent ocean of consciousness within, we come back out into activity with a little more of the silence, energy, creativity and balance—which is the nature of consciousness itself. Having this experience regularly is said to be the basis of maintaining a state of peaceful equanimity within the incessant activity of life—the eye of the hurricane. The usual worries, anxieties and fears that can commonly fill our thoughts fail to grip us so much. Combined with simple living, the regular cultivation of the state of restful alertness is what the ancient sages and yogic masters used as the basis for their spiritual growth. Ultimately, this is what enabled them to live '*in this world, but not of this world,* i.e. to live successfully in the world without being rocked by the fluctuating fortunes of life.

At the conclusion of my instruction, I was recommended to practice my new technique twice a day. I did this diligently, even meditating in football change rooms (that was certainly a challenge!), on planes and in my car. Although I didn't have the same unbounded experience each time, it was always relaxing, enjoyable and highly rejuvenating. Motivated by my experiences, I wanted to learn more about the practice of transcending, and began avidly researching the topic. I discovered that in traditions such as the Vedic tradition of India, transcending the everyday world of thoughts was seen to be the basis of what the spiritual adepts called 'enlightenment'. As the theory went, when we transcend mind, body and senses, we become one with our source. With time, we experience the 'light of God' and some would say, enter the kingdom of heaven. The inner light of consciousness begins to shine more fully, and we naturally begin to radiate that light in our lives. That all seemed light years away from my own experience—at 19 all I cared about was girls and football!—but it sure sounded good.

The more I read, the more I realized that there was a united thread of transcendence linking many of the world's most well-known figures. The great discoveries of scientists such as Einstein, Archimedes and Newton were all accompanied by self-described transcendental experiences. Many scholars suggest that the missing years of Jesus' life were spent in the East transcending his way to higher consciousness. The Buddha was said to have transcended the sufferings of the world in order to gain enlightenment or nirvana during his 40 days under the bodhi tree. The Vedic texts that date back thousands of years detail how the ancient 'rishis' (seers of reality) brought to light the innumerable laws of nature that govern our world, including the principles of Ayurveda contained in this book, through individual and collective transcending.

Despite the impressive history of transcendence, I was also interested to see whether such mental technologies are practical and useful in today's world. Specifically in regard to health, I found that the time honored art of transcending provides a foundation for supporting every area of health and performance. In fact, research studies on TM, which have been conducted at medical schools and universities such as Harvard, Stanford, UCLA and Yale, and reported in the most prestigious scientific journals throughout the world[1], clearly demonstrate the power of transcending. The findings showed that regular transcendence helps everything from reducing blood pressure, stress, anxiety, substance abuse and depression to optimizing brain functioning, increasing self-actualization (the ability to realize more of one's potential) and even promoting higher states of consciousness.[2] Many of today's most widespread diseases, such as heart disease, diabetes and obesity, were also shown to be significantly reduced.[3] My favorite finding, however, was that people who had transcended on a daily basis for more than five years were found to have reduced their biological age, i.e. the actual functional age of their body, by over twelve years.[4] It seemed that while cosmetic creams and potions may help us look good on the outside, transcending provided an even more powerful way to retard the aging process ... from the inside.

One practice, multiple benefits

From a spiritual standpoint, the true importance of transcending is that it allows us to improve the quality of our thinking and behavior in a most natural, effortless way. It is our thoughts and actions which ultimately determine our success in life. While we might know intellectually that we should eat well and exercise regularly, if we are not happy and content within ourselves, history tells us that we will not keep up these healthy practices for long. According to enlightened spiritual teachers throughout time, working at the level of thought or behavior, such as positive thinking or behavioral change, does not represent the ultimate way to progress in life. This is because our thoughts and behaviors are merely by-products of a deeper reality—our level of consciousness. Unless we first enliven the silent field of consciousness, the task of thinking more positively, quitting smoking, eating less junk food, or knowing what work is most suitable for us, will always be difficult. This is why the success of most new diets, fad exercise regimes and self-help programs is usually short-lived. Real change must be made from within. It must be made from the level of consciousness itself.

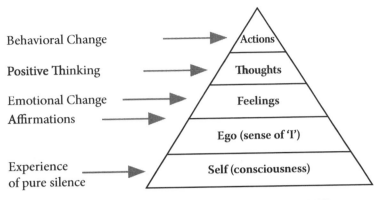

LEAST POWERFUL LEVEL

Behavioral Change ⟶ Actions

Positive Thinking ⟶ Thoughts

Emotional Change ⟶ Feelings
Affirmations ⟶

Ego (sense of 'I')

Experience
of pure silence ⟶ Self (consciousness)

MOST POWERFUL LEVEL

Diagram 5: Effective Change
Trying to change behavior solely on the level of actions, thoughts, or feelings,
is usually hard work and time-consuming (if successful at all). In order
to make behavioral change more immediate and natural, ideally we need to
nourish the most basic level of life—the level of consciousness.

Wise teachers throughout time have declared that the ultimate source of our greatest health and inner contentment does not exist in the outer world of sensory pleasures and 24/7 activity. It resides in the transcendental field of life.

Only by transcending and enlivening our silent inner source can we truly nourish our health and happiness from the deepest level.

Enlivening inner silence—Ideas to help

1. Experience silence daily

   Where possible, try to make some room to hear the music in your life. Look to incorporate one or two 'pause periods' in your day to enjoy some inner silence, e.g.

   i. switch off your car radio, TV or iPod and 'just be' for a while
   ii. say a prayer or do a 'gratitude reflection' in bed at the start or end of the day
   iii. take time to watch a sunrise or sunset occasionally just sit and close your eyes every now and then
   iv. if you ever get the opportunity, try spending 30 minutes, an hour or even half a day in silence.

2. Minimize stress

   Stress severely limits our ability to experience inner silence and transcendence. If you go outside on a cloudy day, you might say, 'Blast, the sun is not out today'. However, the sun would be shining as it always does. It's just that the clouds are blocking your experience of the sun's light and warmth.

   Similarly, too much physiological stress obstructs our ability to naturally experience the light of consciousness shining within us. Appreciate that stress is by far the greatest obstacle to your long-term wellbeing and, wherever possible, reduce or eliminate anything that causes you significant, ongoing stress. Also, incorporate activities into your daily and weekly routine that help prevent stress from accumulating in your life. These might include yoga, music therapy, massage, hobbies, social catch-ups or common relaxation-based meditation practices.

3. Learn how to 'transcend'

   While transcendental experiences can be had on an ad hoc basis (listening to beautiful music, being totally engaged in a passion, etc), learning how to systematically transcend is arguably the single most important thing we can do for our health and wellbeing. If you already do a meditation or relaxation practice that provides good benefits, then certainly continue this. However, if you don't currently transcend on a regular basis, look to add a transcending-based meditation practice such as TM into your daily routine.[a] (I still practice TM and consider it one of the best things I've ever done.)

NOTE: The concept of transcending is not to be confused with today's concept of meditation. These days meditation has largely become a generic term that can apply to anything from focused breathing techniques, visualization or contemplation to listening to the sounds of nature. Some people even call a hobby or exercise their 'meditation'. While all these things, and indeed anything that calms the mind or relaxes the body are to be strongly encouraged, it should be noted that the effects of such practices are quite different from the effects of transcending.

Seed wisdom

As the gardeners of our own tree of life, if we want to do just one thing to strengthen every area of our life, we need to nourish the unseen spiritual part of ourselves—that which lies within.

Ancient sages from India, Tibet, China, Japan, South America and beyond all taught that quietening the mind and experiencing inner silence is the age-old formula for maximizing our success in life. Only by transcending can we take our mind out of stress and into silence. The more we enliven our infinite field of consciousness within, the more we align ourselves with the natural laws of health and cultivate our own inner wisdom (the final wisdom in this book).

By nourishing our silent source, we spontaneously begin to live more in tune with nature's cycles. We naturally desire more health-promoting food and exercise. We gain greater clarity about what relationships and

---

a   TM is taught in nearly every country of the world. Simply look for the Maharishi Mahesh Yogi Transcendental Meditation (TM) center in your nearest city. For the USA, see www.tm.org

vocations most nourish us, and we are better able to negotiate our way through the complexities of modern-day health advice. By 'watering the root' (our non-physical spiritual core), we are better able to 'enjoy the fruit'—better health and success in every area of life.

If you only want to do one thing to promote your health and happiness, transcend and enliven the silent source of all that you are.

Transcend   Transcend   Transcend

Wisdom Seven

First and Foremost, Follow Your Inner Wisdom

The first step in the acquisition of wisdom is silence;
the second listening...
Solomon Ibn Gabriol

The impatient young doctor looked at the woman and said rather matter-of-factly, 'Your breast will need to be removed. We've booked you in for a mastectomy in two weeks. The nurse will explain the rest'. Regardless of how they are said, such words would tear at the heart of any woman. But that was that. The doctor's mind was made up. The decision was made. No further discussion was necessary. The next patient was waiting. The scan shows 'a' so you do 'b'.

Although from a clinical perspective such a diagnosis may have made perfect sense, Georgina wasn't convinced. Having realized that her illness was in no small part related to the fact that she had not followed the subtle signals her body had been giving her over the past few years, she was now acutely aware of the little voice inside her which was screaming at her, 'No, this doesn't need to happen. This is not necessary.' At home that evening, try as she might to rationalize her gut reaction, the nagging little voice became louder and louder. 'This doesn't have to happen. Get a second opinion.' A few days later, Georgina and her partner were sitting in the office of the hospital's senior surgeon. After a short consultation, during which he seemed just as interested in her feelings and trepidations as he was in the scans, he performed his own personal check on Georgina. In his opinion, a full mastectomy wasn't needed at all. A standard lumpectomy, where merely the cancerous tissue is removed, would be fine.

To this day Georgina still has her own breasts. More importantly, what she learnt that day was what many of our wisest ancestors have suggested represents the ultimate wisdom of health.

> Just as important as any authoritative text, healing guru or medical test is the quiet voice inside that whispers to us the truest truths.

Listen up—your body might be telling you something

In the blockbuster movie of 2010, *'Avatar'*, the main character Jake Sully has to learn the ways of the indigenous owners of the land—the Na'vi people. Before anything else, he is first taught to follow the wisdom of his own body. He says, 'I have to trust my body to know what to do.' James Cameron, the director of *'Avatar'*, has said that the Na'vi people were based on various *indigenous cultures* living around the world. Common amongst many of these cultures is the understanding that there is a network of energy and intelligence that flows through all things, including us. We humans are seen as one part of a greater web of life, and the basic goal of life is simply to flow with the unseen intelligence that governs this web. It is understood that we are guided to do this through feedback from our own body. The elders of traditional cultures, aptly known as the *'wisdom keepers'*, suggest that our body's inner wisdoms are messages from our true or higher self—our spirit or soul.

When our spirit enters the earthly plane, it is temporarily housed in a body, often called the 'house' or 'living temple'. It is said that if we keep our temple clean and clear—by observing the wisdoms of health and performing internal cleansing routines (house cleaning)—we are better able to hear our spirit's guiding messages.

In just the last few years, mind-body medicine has begun to reinforce some of these age-old understandings. Just as we help create the chemical environment of our bodies based on our dominant thoughts and emotions (see Wisdom One), the latest research also tells us that the same chemical messengers work the other way. That is, what happens in our bodies on a cellular and even energetic level is constantly being relayed back to our body's central command. We now know, for example, that chemicals produced by our immune system when fighting cancer have receptors in our brains.[1] And it's not just our immune system that relays messages back to us. Our heart, liver, spleen, kidneys, intestines and every other organ are sending back status reports via chemical, electrical, hormonal and vibrational couriers in every moment of our existence.[a]

---

a   For the sake of simplicity we have implied that our body's central command is specifically located in our brain. However, our body's central command (intelligence) is in no way confined to our brains.

Diagram 6: The Body's 24/7 Feedback System

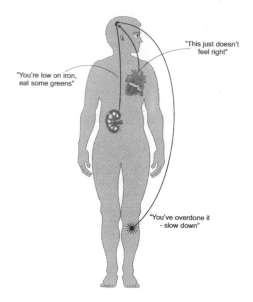

"This just doesn't feel right"

"You're low on iron, eat some greens"

"You've overdone it - slow down"

Of course, we don't need to decipher these complex chemical or electrical codes. Mother Nature delivers these signals in a far simpler and more tangible way—via our gut feelings and subtle intuition. Through what's known as *psychoneuroimmunology* or PNI, modern science is now confirming what the traditional sciences have said for millennia: our gut feelings are far more than just feelings, they are physical realities. When we are joyful, our hearts don't just feel joy emotionally, they feel joy 'physically'. If we are angry, our livers feel physically 'angry'. Our stomachs can feel physically anxious and our bladders can feel physically fearful. This may explain the phenomenon of when we 'just know' that something isn't right. We often say, 'I just don't feel right, I know something is wrong'. Conversely, after having a serious illness, at some point in their recovery many people have been known to suddenly remark, 'It's gone, I just know it's gone. I can feel it'.

The practical implication of all this, as taught by Vedic masters, ancient Mayans and generations of Aborigines through to the great lamas of Tibet, is that our gut feelings are our inner healing signposts. Like the

GPS navigation systems in our cars, our subtle whims and intangible emotions act as guides in helping us to maintain balance and joy. Feeling good doesn't just 'feel good', it is an indication that things are good. Conversely, feeling that something 'isn't quite right' is usually the first sign that it isn't. If a group of cancer cells are dividing somewhere in our body, the message we get might be in the form of a subtle desire for more rest or to eat a certain type of food. If things progress to the point of disease, it might be a not so subtle feeling of needing to leave a stressful job or to heal a toxic relationship. We can dismiss these feelings as impractical, or reject them because modern science cannot quantify them and thus considers them unscientific, but all time-honored natural health sciences suggest that they are the most accurate and trustworthy diagnostic tools we have.

Sonia Esquivel certainly thinks following our body's internal messages is wise. Four years ago, she had a hysterectomy. The operation followed a long period of haemorrhages that left her dramatically anaemic. A year after the operation she was still constantly tired, which in turn made her quite depressed. She would come back from work and want to go to sleep at 6pm. She picks up the story:

> I went to the doctor and after blood tests were performed, he told me I still had the same levels of anaemia. He recommended a diet high in iron and suggested the possibility of using supplements if this did not work. However, something inside me knew that this was not the answer. I had always had a very healthy diet and was basically already eating what he recommended. It just didn't seem right. What I actually felt, a sort of 'gut feeling' if you like, was that I needed to exercise more. If I put my body in motion, it would need more oxygen and in this way it would be forced to produce more red blood cells. That is what I now believe happened. I started by riding to work once a week and built that up to where I now ride every day. My anaemia has disappeared, my blood pressure is perfect, I feel great, and my blood tests, as my doctor put it, *'are those of a 12 year old!'*

Animals certainly don't need the latest peer-reviewed research studies or Harvard-trained professors to guide them to better balance. In the animal world there is a concept known as '*nutritional wisdom*'. This explains how animals naturally seek out particular foods (medicines) to cure themselves of illness. CSIRO scientists have even undertaken research based on the ability of sheep to choose foods that meet their nutritional needs. They also believe that sick sheep know how to 'self-medicate' by gravitating to plants that help them get well. Interestingly, some pioneering medical practitioners are now even suggesting that we (the patients) may be our own best doctors, and that our intuition should be used to help them most accurately diagnose and treat us. In an article on clinical intuition, Glyn Brokensha, former Senior Lecturer in the Medical Education Unit at the University of Adelaide, says, 'Most patients have a wealth of this (intuitive) experience. This is not generally in the domains of clinical knowledge and skill, but in their own experience they are 'de facto' experts!'[2] In Ayurveda and other traditional medical systems, doctors were trained to pay just as much if not more attention to a patient's own feelings and intuitions about their illness as they were to any physical signs and symptoms.

Although being better able to diagnose problems once they have manifested is a good thing, the deeper reality in all this is that our bodies are likely to send us feedback, well before disease manifests, as to how we might prevent illness-creating imbalances from developing in the first place. This is not just in regard to serious illness but even in common, everyday situations. Sydney's Barbara Groom cites an example of the simple, everyday bodily wisdoms we often fail to follow.

I recently found myself sneezing frequently as well as having a runny nose. Like many people, this is usually a precursor to a really bad head cold for me. However, as I had a long-standing arrangement to travel interstate in the next few days, becoming ill was not an option. I've learnt over the years that when I start getting sick, it is my body telling me something. Instead of soldiering on and taking medication, I knew I had to stop running around and take it easy for a couple of days. I made sure I got to bed extra early, slept in a bit later, avoided the gym or any over-exertion, and tried to work in a short afternoon rest. My symptoms got no worse, the cold never eventuated, and by the time of my trip I was feeling much clearer and more energetic.

> The more science looks at our body's internal communication systems, the more it is confirming the wisdom of our forefathers.
>
> By tuning in more to our 'inner healing messengers', the ancients suggest that we can avert much sickness before it even begins.

Inner wisdom exercises

1. Every now and then stop what you are doing, close your eyes, and put your attention on your body. Ask yourself the following questions (or any that are more pertinent to you) and 'listen in' for the answers.

   - How is my posture?
   - Do I have any tension, stiffness or pain anywhere in my body? If so, why might this be?
   - Am I hungry?
   - Am I tired?
   - Is my breathing deep and relaxed or short and shallow? Why is that?
   - When I think of my work or primary daily activity, what do I feel—excitement, pleasure, indifference, unease, anxiety, stress?
   - What is the best thing I can do for my health right now?

2. Go for a walk and consciously notice the things around you. Be grateful for what nourishes your life—the sun, the air, the trees, other people. Getting your attention off yourself and becoming more conscious of the health-promoting gifts around you will help strengthen your connection to your spirit and amplify your inner wisdom.[3]

Going beyond the confusions of conventional health advice

The intuitive mind is a sacred gift. The rational mind its faithful servant.

Albert Einstein

In addition to helping prevent health problems manifesting or escalating, the other great benefit of consulting our inner doctor is in helping us avoid much of the complexity and confusion of modern-day health advice. Should we or shouldn't we eat meat? Is dairy healthy or harmful? Is high or low intensity exercise best? Is getting out in the sun sinful or sagacious?

In contrast to the almost unlimited number of experts, magazines, TV shows and advertisements telling us what's healthy today, the most heavily researched groups of long-living people have had a complete lack of such advice. Older Okinawans, Vilcabambans, Sardinians, Hunzans and Abkhasians, as well as vibrant, healthy elders from centuries past, never had self-help gurus, celebrity experts or cutting-edge research findings to guide them to better health. All they had was their own observational and bodily wisdom. This 'self-knowledge', as it was known, is what forms the foundation of the Eastern health approaches. Self-knowledge is based on the understanding that our bodies possess their own intrinsic knowing or 'inner wisdom'. It was appreciated that only by developing this internal wisdom can we truly go beyond the endless dichotomies of health and know what is right for us as individuals.

The highest truths of health and happiness resonate within us.

When we hear or experience a universal truth or what is true for us, every cell of our body tingles. Every molecule of our DNA sings. We don't need science or some external authority to confirm it. In our heart of hearts we 'just know' what is right and what is not.

In contrast to the Eastern world view, which seeks to satisfy both the head and the heart, our Western approach is largely based on intellectual knowledge. Intellectual knowledge resides firmly in the rational, logical mind and comes in the form of books, expert opinion and scientific discoveries. These are all wonderful sources of knowledge and can certainly be used to guide us to better health. However, as such knowledge is often based on individual opinion, isolated aspects of health, or reality from one particular point of view, it can also create much confusion and misunderstanding.

On the day I was writing this, the main segment on the leading national morning television program was how a 'new scientific study' had shown that formula milk was just as good as breast milk for newborn babies. This clicked into gear the old chestnut of 'Is breast best?' As the day proceeded, media and experts from every corner of the country weighed into the debate. Leading researchers and eminent authorities from near and far were interviewed. Some detailed how formula milk was the nutritional equivalent of breast milk. Others put forward the 'breast is best' argument. The result was a pot pourri of science, personal opinion, vested interests, and what no good debate should be without—quotes from Joe or Jo Public. 'A friend of mine had her baby on formula from day dot and she got straight A's in high school.' 'I breastfed my four kids until they were eighteen and now they are all Olympic champions!' I'm joking here but I think you get the idea. In the end, I'm sure all that was accomplished was that any nursing mother watching or listening would have felt totally confused and utterly bewildered. You could just hear the collective sigh of mothers across the country struggling to breastfeed—'Is it (breastfeeding) really worth the effort?'

Now, I obviously have next to no first-hand experience in this area (apart from almost 40 years ago!), but difficulties of breastfeeding aside, do we really need such debates? Isn't there an intrinsic knowing within every mother that regardless of any research, breastfeeding their newborn is without equal? If we take a step back from the so-called 'science', do we not appreciate that breastfeeding is much more than specific nutrients in breast milk, whether or not they are similar to those in an artificial formula? Surely, breastfeeding is a holistic amalgam of not only nutrition but also love. Surely, it is about the bonding of mother and baby, and the flood of healing biochemistry created when the two unite in the greatest of all intimacies. (What love-based chemicals in breast milk can science not detect?) Surely, breastfeeding is about a connection so powerful there are not words to describe it, let alone scientific instruments to measure it. This is not to denigrate in any way the many women who would love to breastfeed but simply cannot for one reason or another, or those where the stress of doing so means they understandably choose not to.[b] I personally believe that when we appreciate the physical effects of our emotions, a baby fed formula milk by a happy, stress-free mother may in fact be far better off than a baby breastfed by a mother who is enduring immense pain or discomfort. However, if we get to the point where we start believing there is little or no difference between breast milk and formula, it is a sign that we have distanced ourselves too far from the commonsense wisdoms of health.

The point here is not to diminish the benefits of modern science. I've used many examples of it throughout this book. However, it is in the nature of modern scientific method that there will always be times where the science is unclear or inconclusive. Ironically, the overload of (often conflicting) scientific health information in today's world is more likely to obstruct rather than promote our optimal health. This is because we get so brainwashed into thinking that the key to health is in the next big scientific breakthrough or the revolutionary new weight-loss diet that we forget that the simplest, most profound truths about health and healing are literally shouting at us from within. Sometimes we need to simply stop accepting everything we hear and start consulting a higher wisdom ... our inner wisdom. The following are a couple of good examples of people who have followed their inner wisdom to better health.

---

b   It may be noted that problems relating to breastfeeding are often usually experienced far less in traditional cultures, where time-tested nursing wisdom is passed down from mother (or grandmother) to daughter.

Miriam Petrakis from Sydney was going through heavy periods. She went to her local GP, who suggested (if you can believe it), 'Why don't you have a hysterectomy?' Miriam didn't think that this was such a good idea but went and had a blood test, pap smear and various scans. The results were all fine, so she then went to see a gynaecologist. The gynaecologist told her it was quite normal that this was happening and she could be just going through 'the change of life'—even though her blood tests didn't say so. It was recommended she could either have a day procedure that 'wouldn't necessarily help the problem', try the contraceptive pill or take Naprogesic—a non-steroidal anti-inflammatory which had always made her feel bloated and sick!

Understandably, Miriam wasn't too keen about any of these ideas. She says, 'After the visit, I wasn't happy. Something wasn't right and I knew there must be a simpler answer to all this (her inner wisdom speaking). Instead of going down that track, I felt to contact a naturopath and I began adjusting my diet and taking herbal medicine. In just a few months, things improved remarkably, and I have had no need to consider the other interventions. I have always felt that you don't simply remove something if it is not working, you have to strengthen the organs that are weak. It might take longer, but it's worth it.'

Sixteen years ago, Theo, a seminar client of mine, had a lower back problem that was so severe that for several months, he had to sleep on the lounge room floor. The tiniest movement resulted in immense pain. He had gone to many doctors and specialists and recalled the last specialist telling him that he would never jog again. For someone who had been a jogger for many years, this news was not taken well. There was recommended to take it easy and only do low-level non-strenuous exercise. He did this for two to three months without any improvement. Theo continues the story. 'Something within me told me that I had to try something else—that the less I did, the more my body would become weaker not stronger. I decided to take things into my own hands and began a steady exercise regime of walking and swimming. I remember that this was initially somewhat painful, but overall it felt good. After a few months, I was at the point where I began to jog again. Following this, whenever I got a bad back, instead of doing less activity, I would put up with the initial discomfort and head out for a jog. In most cases, I'd be pain free within a few days.' (Interestingly, although it used to be standard practice to advise total rest for most back pain, in recent years things have come almost full circle. Now moderate activity is often recommended as the best way to assist many types of back pain.)

The above examples, as with all the case studies cited in this chapter, are in no way intended to suggest that we should devalue good medical advice. It is just that we also need to honor our own intuitions. Make use of doctors' and health practitioners' wealth of clinical knowledge and experience, but also speak up and have your own gut feelings heard.

> Our clearest and most profound insights into what we need for health and happiness rarely come from outside sources, they come from the infinite field of intuition deep within.
>
> Rather than being solely reliant on science or external experts, we do well not to overlook the sage-like wisdoms that guide us from within. This is what enlightened medicine men and women throughout time have suggested we pay most attention to.

Using your inner wisdom—Ideas to help

1. First and foremost, appreciate that while the ideas presented here may sound simple, for most of us, tuning in to our higher wisdoms is by no means easy. (I often feel a divine impulse to spend the weekend sitting on the couch watching football. However, I am informed by my partner—in no uncertain terms—that my inner wisdom requires major corrective surgery!) Seriously, while enlightened spiritual sages might spontaneously follow the highest wisdoms of health, for most of us, learning to hear, let alone trust, our subtle intuitions can be a challenge. The key is to just start the process and begin listening to your body's internal messages. Like going to the gym for the first time, start with simple, everyday things (like light weights) and gradually build up to more important issues (heavy weights).

2. Every time you hear the results of a new scientific study or read health recommendations of any sort (including those in this book), don't simply accept them. First, run things past your inner doctor. Ask yourself, 'Does this feel right?'

3. Cultivate the long forgotten and commonly underused 'wisdom of commonsense'. It's amazing how often we don't do what makes simple sense, e.g. eating an orange or some strawberries instead of swallowing vitamin C pills.

4. Appreciate that if something is in harmony with your own personal laws of nature, it will resonate with you. You will feel it in your bones and in your heart. Learn to trust and follow that feeling and be wary of the opposite feeling, i.e. that nagging feeling that something 'just isn't right'.

5. If you are still feeling confused, do what the ancients did in developing their time-tested wisdoms. Traditionally, cultures without access to billion-dollar microscopes, x-ray machines or other technologies gained great wisdom from the simple science of observation. If you are not sure how much wheat or dairy foods are best for your constitution, eat more or less of them and 'observe' the results. How do you feel? Do some exer-

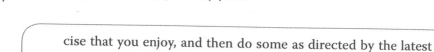

cise that you enjoy, and then do some as directed by the latest fat-burning guru. Which innately feels right for you?

6. Meditate regularly. As discussed in Wisdom Six, meditation, or more particularly transcending, cultures our level of inner silence. Ultimately, it is only through experiencing more inner silence that we heighten our ability to 'just know' what is right for us.

Examples of when you might use your inner wisdom

1. When choosing a doctor, natural healthcare practitioner, dietician or personal trainer. Don't just go on credentials or convenience, also consult your gut feeling about whether they feel right for you.
2. When someone is trying to sell you a new health product or to convince you of a new eating, exercise or success formula.
3. If you are dealing with a major health issue and feel overwhelmed by conflicting advice about what is best for you to do.

Laurel's story

Ironically, one of the best illustrations of the profound health improvements we can receive by tuning into our body's inner wisdom, comes from my wonderful book editor, Laurel. I think Laurel's personal story is an inspiring and beautiful example of the fundamental importance of this final wisdom of health. (Laurel knew it all, it's just that like many of us, the 'busyness' of life got in the way.)

When I started editing this book, I was in a fairly depleted state. My long-standing nasal and sinus allergies were only 'under control' because I took one 24-hour antihistamine every 36 hours (as I had for years). Without this, I would sneeze uncontrollably and had itchy, swollen nasal passages at all times. As my workload in my stressful teaching job reached a peak towards the end of last term, the 36-hour window retreated towards 24 hours before I had to take another antihistamine. I was always tired, especially on waking, and then ear infections flared up, which four visits to the ear specialist over five weeks would not settle. They were extremely itchy, inflamed, oozing and closed up, so my hearing was limited. I sensed that the fungal ear infections were allergy-related, but felt I had nowhere to turn with doctors in that area. Eighteen months earlier, I had completed three years of desensitisation injections with an allergy specialist, and after extensive tests had been pronounced 'allergy-free', although my nose symptoms were still very much present!

Reading through this book reminded me of some of the basics of good health that I had moved away from in my life. This included the idea of listening to my body's own wisdom. I'd been working too hard and compensating for the pressure with comfort foods like chocolate and lattes. Although I had believed that I couldn't give up my daily coffee habit, I now 'knew' (through my inner wisdom) that I had to 'clear out everything'. In one go, I gave up coffee, sweets and all dairy products, as well as the antihistamines. I also felt a strong need to meditate, and my mind 'fell into it' whenever I could over a long weekend. It was a huge relief to my physiology. Since then, I have taken charge by approaching my work in a more measured way and initiating a comprehensive 'detox' diet. These days, my health is my absolute first priority. I have not taken or needed to take a single antihistamine for three months. My ears cleared up after one-and-a-half weeks, and since then I have barely felt any of the ear itchiness which was always there for fifteen years. My body and mind feel much more at peace, as if a burden has been removed from them.

Laurel finished by saying how the book simply reminded her of what she already knew in herself. This was my favorite part because it is so true for all of us. We know these things, we just need to reconnect with them and remind ourselves how infinitely wise our own bodies are.

Seed wisdom

What we seek is not outside ourselves ... It is so close, we overlook it.

Lama Surya Das[4]

Most of us don't know we are going to have a heart attack until we do. We don't know we have cancer until the test results show it. But what if our bodies are telling us whether or not we are heading in the direction of ill health well in advance?

The likely truth is that our bodies are doing that in every moment of our existence and they're doing it with more wisdom, more accuracy and more immediacy than any medical scan or test may ever do. It is only when we learn to trust the quiet voice of wisdom inside us that we begin to access the deeper wisdoms that guide our lives. It is this inner wisdom which is our highest wisdom.

Ultimately, everything in this book is at best a basic guide. Don't follow any of it based solely on science or what I say. The only true way to know what is right for you at any particular time is to listen to, and trust, your own body—your inner doctor. Sure, eating light at night might be good, but what is light for you? Sure, it's good to go to bed early, but isn't celebrating with friends or working on something that inspires you with a greater purpose also healthy? And who can tell you how much food you need, when you are tired, or what type of work inspires you? Not your spouse. Not any doctor. Not any coach. Not me. Only you can. Only your infinitely intelligent mind, body and spirit ... if you listen to it.

> Consult the many experts and resources that can help you towards your higher health, but first and foremost, tune in to the divine, inner wisdoms of health that are being whispered to you in every moment of your existence.

Epilogue

Keep It Simple—Happiness is No. 1

You've been provided with a perfect body to house your soul for a few brief moments in eternity. So regardless of its size, shape, color, or any imagined infirmities, you can honor the temple that houses you by eating healthfully, exercising, listening to your body's needs, and treating it with dignity and love.

Dr Wayne Dyer

Art Brownstein tells a marvelous story by the legendary healer Dr Bernie Siegel, in his excellent book *'Extraordinary Healing'*. [1]

A man ran six miles every day for 25 years. He never went to parties, he never went to bed after 10pm, never drank or smoked, and was a vegetarian. One day, he suddenly died. He was so upset by this sudden turn of events that when he got to the Pearly Gates he went straight up to God and demanded an explanation for this apparent injustice.

'What the hell are you doing, God?' the man asked. 'I've run every day for the past 25 years, never touched alcohol or tobacco, gone to bed early, and eaten only vegetables. I've worked hard my whole life just to remain healthy and live long, and you had to spoil everything by bringing me here. What's your point in doing this?'

'My point is that you basically blew it!' God said. 'You forgot to have fun and enjoy your life, which were the reasons why you were created!' God went on, 'And since you failed to learn your lessons this time, I'm sending you back to Hell for an attitude adjustment!'

'What will I do there?' queried the man.

'For starters, you'll have to run six miles every day, go to bed before 10pm each night, and eat only vegetables,' God declared. He continued, 'Next time, try to enjoy your life, and come back when your attitude is a little better!'

I think this story beautifully sums up one of the most important lessons of health. It's more important to be happy than to be 'healthy'. While I hope you found some of the points in this book helpful, do not feel you have to do them all in order to be healthy. Despite the commonsense wisdom of many of our wise predecessors, regularly doing everything that promotes good health can be a strain in our modern world. With our busy lives, the secrets of good health may be simple, but they are not always easy. I certainly don't pretend to enjoy perfect health (two concussions and the seeds of arthritis from 15 years' playing football have seen to that!). Nor am I able to follow all of the wisdoms of good health all of the time. If you are a single parent or a working parent with two or three young kids, I can only imagine how challenging incorporating many of the ideas recommended here would be at times. The point is, more important than 'doing all the right things' is 'doing what's right for you'. While it's good to follow a healthy lifestyle, never do it to the point of compromising your enjoyment of life.

Last but not least, at the deepest level of who you are, know that the true secrets to health and happiness do not require a Masters degree in Science. They are not to be found under a microscope or inside a petri dish. The real keys are astoundingly simple. They have existed since the dawn of time and are forever whispering to you (shouting at you) from within. First and foremost, do what nourishes your heart, and most of the time live in tune with the eternal cycles of Mother Nature, eat natural foods, move your body in ways that bring you joy, connect to the sun, fresh air, clean water and the earth, experience some inner silence each day, and begin to listen in to, and trust, the little voice inside you guiding you along your way. It really doesn't get any more complicated than that.

In five, ten or twenty years' time, you won't even hear about things such as the Atkins Diet, Glycemic Index or any of the other innumerable fads that fill our bookstores and TV programs today. They will have been replaced with a new wave of catchy, marketing savvy programs and products, based on isolated aspects of health, promising you the next 'revolutionary' way to great (and quick) health. However, in ten, twenty and even a thousand years, the unchanging, immutable principles of health that are forever governing your mind, body and spirit, and have been followed by the world's healthiest people throughout time, will be functioning just as they always have been.

The real keys to lifelong health and wellness are nothing that you don't already know—if not consciously, then at least intuitively. If you haven't already done so, may you re-embrace the simple wisdoms of health and enjoy a wonderfully happy life.

Yours in good health
Mark Bunn

Acknowledgements

To Mum and Dad, thank you for everything. You started me on this journey and have been the foundation for everything I enjoy in life. I love you both so much.

A big thank you also to all of the following:

To big brother Paul and big sister Claire—for whatever wisdom you imparted in between harassing your poor little brother!

To dear Lorna, my wonderful teacher, inspiration and friend—for your limitless knowledge, unbounded heart and eternal guidance.

To the great Andrew Stenberg—for all your heart, soul and wisdom that is in this book.

To darling Aunt Lois and the great dog-whispering Tara King—for your initial reading and improving of my very 'rough' manuscripts.

To Laurel Acton, editor extraordinaire, and Diane Davie, the Pitta perfect proofreader—thanks for your invaluable contributions. You have given so much more than what was asked.

To Leon Nacsen—for your generous spirit and wise counsel regarding 'all things book publishing'.

To the self-publishing maestro, Dale Beaumont—for the inspiration to self publish and for the great wisdom on how to do it successfully. You rock!

To the great Raamon Newman—embodiment of Ram—for your inspiration and ongoing support in getting the book out to many more people around the world than would otherwise have occurred.

To Sherry Strong, Cyndi O'Meara, and Karen Coulson—for your wonderful nutritional wisdom.

To Mia Dalby-Ball—for your generous spirit in passing on some of the timeless wisdoms of our dear indigenous brothers and sisters.

To the many other authors and researchers who have brought to light many great wisdoms of natural health. With special mention to John Robbins, Sally Beare, Don Tolman, Krispin Sullivan and Dr William Grant.

And last but not least, to Maharishi Mahesh Yogi, who more than any other introduced me to the essential wisdoms of health, and whose profound knowledge forms the foundation of much of this book.

References

Part I—*The wisdom of wisdoms*

1. Extract reproduced with thanks to Sally Beare, *The Live Longer Diet*, 2003, Piatkus (Little, Brown Book Group).

2. Beare, S. *The Live Longer Diet*, 2003, Piatkus (Little, Brown Book Group).

3. Robbins, J. *Healthy at 100*. 2006. Published by Random House.

4. Campbell, TC. Campbell, TM. *The China Study*. 2006. BenBella Books.

5. Ibid. pp 71. Cited from Doll, R. and Peto, R. 'The causes of cancer: Quantitative estimates of avoidable risks of cancer in the United States today.' *J Natl Cancer Inst*. 1981. 66. pp 1192-1265.

Part II—*The seven wisdoms*

Wisdom One

1. I am not sure where this quote originally came from but I came upon it courtesy of my good friend and inspirational teacher Andrew Stenberg. It may well have come from Andrew himself but he couldn't quite remember—his brain is so full of great things.

2. Tolman, D. *Farmacist Desk Reference*. 2005. Benaquista Publishing Inc. pp 86.

3. Faith R.E., Murgo A.J., Plontikoff N.P. Interactions between the immune system and the nervous system. *Stress and immunity*. 1991. CRC, Boca Raton. pp 287-303.

4 & 5. View the groundbreaking work by Dr. Candace Pert—a pioneer in the field of pyschoneuroimmunology and author of books including 'Molecules of Emotion'. As a side note, in her latest book, *Everything You Need to Know to Feel Go(o)d*, Dr Pert discusses how our emotional communication networks are really more a matter of underlying physics than they are physical chemistry or biology.

6.   i) A typical example of such studies is Medalie, JH. Goldbourt, U. Angina Pectoris among 10,000 men. II. Psychosocial and other risk factors as evidenced by multivariate analysis of a five year incidence study. *American Journal of Medicine.* 1976:60(6): pp 910-921.

   ii) Also see 7. below.

7.   Tanne, D. Goldbourt, U. Medalie, JH. Perceived Family Difficulties and Prediction of 23-Year Stroke Mortality among Middle-Aged Men *Cerebrovascular Diseases.* 2004:18(4):277-282.

8.   Davidson, KW. Mostofsky, E. and Whang, W. Don't Worry, Be Happy: Positive Affect and Reduced 10-year Incident Coronary Heart Disease: The Canadian Nova Scotia Health Survey. *European Heart Journal,* Feb 17, 2010.

9.   Strathearn, L. Li, J. Fonagy, P. Montague, PR. What's in a Smile? Maternal Brain Responses to Infant Facial Cues. *Paediatrics,* 122 (1) July 2008. pp 40-51.

10.   Wellbeing Index Survey from Australian Unity—Survey 2; Report 2—'Does money buy happiness' and 'The state of contentment'. December 2001. See Executive Summary Notes.

11.   Koch, T. Power, C. Kralik, D. 100 Years Old—24 Australian Centenarians Tell Their Stories. 2005. Penguin Group. pp 6.

12.   Monroe, CM. The Effects of Therapeutic Touch on Pain. *Journal of Holistic Nursing,* 2009. Vol. 27, No. 2, pp 85-92.

13.   With thanks to www.indiaoz.com

14.   Brown, G.W. and Harris, T.O. Social origins of depression: A study of psychiatric disorder in women. 1978. London: Tavistock.

15.   Eng, Patricia M; Rimm, Eric B; Fitzmaurice, Garrett; Kawachi, Ichiro. Social Ties and Change in Social Ties in Relation to Subsequent Total and Causespecific Mortality and Coronary Heart Disease Incidence in Men. 2002. *American Journal of Epidemiology.* 155(8): pp 700-709.

16.   Fowler JH, Christakis NA. Dynamic spread of happiness in a large social network: longitudinal analysis over 20 years in the Framingham Heart Study. *BMJ.* 2008 Dec 4:337:a2338.

17. Solomon, G. and Moos, R. Psychological Aspects of Response to Treatment in Rheumatoid Arthritis', *General Practitioner*. 1965. Dec. Vol 32, no. 6. pp 113-19.

18. Ranga Rama K. George, L. Pieper, C. Jiang, W. Arias, R. Look, A. O'Connor, C. Depression and social support in elderly patients with cardiac disease. *American Heart Journal*. Sept 1998. 136(3): pp 491-495.

19. Lawlor, R. 'Voices of the First Day—Awakening in the Aboriginal Dreamtime'. 1991. Inner Traditions International. pp 242.

    * With great thanks to Robert Lawlor and his book for much of the knowledge relating to the Australian aborigines.

20. Ibid (Lawlor). pp 244.

21. Halsell, G. Los Viejos. pp150-51. * With thanks to John Robbins. HealThat 100 for the original reference.

22. Leaf, A. 'Every Day Is a Gift When You Are Over 100'. *National Geographic*. Jan 1973. Vol 143 (1). pp113.

23. With thanks to John Robbins, *Healthy at 100*. 2006. Published by Random House.

24. Crooks VC, et al. Social network, cognitive function, and dementia incidence among elderly women. *Am J Public Health*. July 2008:98(7) pp 12211227.

25. Berkman, LF. Syme, SL. Social networks, host resistance, and mortality. *American Journal of Epidemiology*. 1979:109. pp 186-204.

26. Study awaiting publishing. Contact study author Dr Rebecca Johnson via http://rechai.missouri.edu/

27. Thoits PA, Hewitt LN. Volunteer work and well-being. *Journal of Health and Social Behavior*. 2001. 42: pp 115-131.

28. i) Greenfield, E.A and Marks, N.F. Formal Volunteering as a Protective Factor for Older Adults. Psychological Well-Being. *The Journals of Gerontology*. 2004. Series B. 59(5): pp S258-S264.

    ii) Musick MA, Wilson J. Volunteering and depression: The role of psychological and social resources in different age groups. *Social Science and Medicine*. 2003:56: pp 259-69.

iii) Arnstein P, Vidal M, Wells-Federman C, et al. From chronic pain patient to peer: benefits and risks of volunteering. *Pain Management Nursing*. 2002:3: pp 94-103.

29. *Story recounted on* speaking on *'You Can Heal your Life'* (Louise Hay) DVD. 2007. Hay House, Inc. Gay Hendricks is a bestselling *author* and co-founder of The *Spiritual Cinema Circle*.

30. Emoto, M. *'The Miracle of Water'* 2007. Atria Books & Beyond Words Publishing.

31. To contact Numeralla Public School regarding their 'make someone's day' program, email numeralla-p.school@det.nsw.edu.au

32. There have numerous studies on the benefits of optimism. For the beneficial effects of optimism on psychological and physical well-being as well as how optimism might allow people to cope with stress more effectively, see

i) Scheier, MF. Carver, CS. Effects of optimism on psychological and physical well-being: Theoretical overview and empirical update. *Cognitive Therapy and Research*. Apr 1992. Vol 16(2).

For how optimism is associated with improved general health, vitality, mental health and reduced bodily pain, see

ii) Achat, H. Kawachi, I. Spiro, A. DeMolles, DA. and Sparrow, D. Optimism and depression as predictors of physical and mental health functioning: The Normative Aging Study. *Annals of Behavioral Medicine*. June 2000. Vol 22(2).

33. For one of many studies on the great longevity of Sardinians, see Deiana, L. Ferrucci, L. Pes, GM. Carru, C. Delitala, G. Ganau, A. Mariotti. S. Nieddu, A. Pettinato, S., Putzu, P. Franceschi. C. Baggio, G. AKEntAnnos. The Sardinia Study of Extreme Longevity. *Aging Clin Exp Res*. 1999;11(3): pp 142-9.

34. Some of the general insights into Sardinian life are from John Hodgman's terrific article, 'How to Live Forever—Secrets of longevity from the island of 100 year old men'. Sept 2005. *Readers Digest*.

35. Leaf, A. 'Every Day Is a Gift When You Are Over 100'. *National Geographic*. Jan 1973. Vol 143 (1). pp 111-12.

Wisdom Two

1. i) Halberg, F. Implications of Biological Rhythms for Clinical Practice, in Krieger, DT. Hughes, JC. (Eds), *Neuroendocrinology;* Sunderland, MA: Sinauer Associates, 1980. pp 109-119; and

    ii) Halberg, F. Haus, E. Cardoso, SS. Schieving, LE. Kuhl, JFW. Shiotsuka, R. Rosene, G. Pauley, JE. Runge, W. Spalding, JR. Lee, JK, Good, RA. Toward a Chronotherapy of Neoplasia: Tolerance of Treatment Depends on Host Rhythms. *Experientia.* August 15, 1973. Basel; 29:909-934.

    * The above references as well as the connection between heart attacks and time of day, were taking from Wallace, RK. *Physiology of Consciousness.* 1993, MIU Press.

2. Sánchez, CL. et al. The possible role of human milk nucleotides as sleep inducers. *Nutritional Neuroscience.* 2009:12(1):2.

3. From an article by Megan Fellman—science and engineering editor at Northwestern University. Study details are; Arble, DM. Bass, J. Laposky, AD. Vitaterna, MH. And Turek, FW. Circadian Timing of Food Intake Contributes to Weight Gain. *Obesity.* 17, 1 November 2009. pp 2100–2102.

4. These cultures include those studied by Alexander Leaf, namely the Hunzans, Vilcabambans, Abkhasians and Okinawans. Other rural cultures in places such as Japan, China, India, North and South America and other places where the incidence of Western diseases have been low, have also generally gone to sleep early in the night cycle.

5. Alimentazione, Nutrizione, Invecchiamento; 2a Campodimele Conference, Obiettivo Longevita (Rome: Edizioni L. Pozzi, 1995).

    * With thanks to Sally Beare, 'The Live longer Diet'. 2003. Piatkus (Little, Brown Book Group). pp 24.

6. Straif, K. Baan, R. Grosse, Y. Secretan, B. El Ghissassi, F. Bouvard, V. Altieri, A. Benbrahim-Tallaa, L. Cogliano, V. on behalf of the WHO International Agency for Research on Cancer Monograph Working GroupCarcinogenicity of Shift-work, Painting, and Fire-fighting. *The Lancet Oncology,* Dec 2007. Vol 8(12). pp 1065–1066.

    * Also, IARC. *IARC monographs on the evaluation of carcinogenic risks to humans.* Preamble. Lyon, France: International Agency for Research on Cancer, 2006.

7. Due to the overwhelming number of relevant studies, no single study is given here. For a range of studies on the subject go to www.pubmed.com and search for 'shift work and disease risk'.

8. Studies include:

Heart disease:

i) Najib, T. Ayas, MD. et al, A Prospective Study of Sleep Duration and Coronary Heart Disease in Women, *Archives of Internal Medicine.* Jan 27, 2003. v. 163, n. 2.

ii) Gnagwisch et al. Short Sleep Duration as a Risk Factor for Hypertension: Analyzes of the First National Health and Nutrition Examination Survey. *Hypertension* 2006;47. pp 833-839.

Breast cancer:

Davis, S. Night Shift Work, Light at Night, and Risk of Breast Cancer. *Journal of the National Cancer Institute.* Oct 17 2001: Vol. 93 (20) pp 15571562.

Autoimmune disorders including rheumatoid arthritis (inflammation):

Irwin, M. Wang, M. Ribeiro, D. Jin Cho, H. Olmstead, R. Crabb Breen, E. Martinez-Maza, O. Cole, S. Sleep Loss Activates Cellular Inflammatory Signaling. *Biological Psychiatry.* 15 Sept 2008. Vol 64(6). pp 538-540.

Weight gain (obesity):

i) Knutson, K. Van Cauter, E. Associations between Sleep Loss and Increased Risk of Obesity and Diabetes. *Ann. N. Y. Acad. Sci.* 2008; 1129: pp 287-304.

ii) Taveras et al. Short Sleep Duration in Infancy and Risk of Childhood Overweight. *Arch Pediatr Adolesc Med* 2008; 162: pp 305-311.

iii) Patel, SR. et al. The Association between Sleep Duration and Obesity in Older Adults. *Int J Obes* (Lond). Dec 2008;32(12): pp 1825-34.

Diabetes:

i) see reference i) under Weight Gain (obesity) above.

ii) Van Cauter, E. Ryden, AM. Mander, BA. Knutson, K et al. Role of sleep duration and quality in the risk and severity of type 2 diabetes mellitus. *Archives of Internal Medicine.* Sept 18, 2006. Vol 166: pp 1768-1774.

iii) Tasali, E. Leproult, R. Ehrmann, D. Van Cauter, E. Slow-wave sleep and the risk of type 2 diabetes in humans. *Proceedings of the National Academy of Science, 2008 105:1044-1049; published online before print.*

iv) Spiegel et al. Sleep loss: A Novel Risk Factor for Insulin Resistance and Type 2 diabetes. *J Appl Physiol.* Nov. 2005; 99(5): pp 2008-2019.

ADHD and behavioral problems in children:

Owens, JA. Maxim, R. Nobile, C. et al. Parental and Self-report of Sleep in Children wiThattention-deficit hyperactivity disorder. *Arch Pediatr Adolesc Med.* 2000:154: pp 549–555.

9. Ruckart, PZ. & Burgess, PA. Human Error and Time of Occurrence in Hazardous Material Events in Mining and Manufacturing. *Journal of Hazardous Materials.* Apr 11 2007: Vol 142(3). pp 747-753.

10. My apologies and acknowledgement to any author who has similarly used this analogy. I am sure it has been used before but cannot remember where. If it should be noted that it has previously been used, please let me know and I will be more than happy to make full acknowledgement in future editions of this book.

11. Examples include;

i) Hayashi, M. Motoyoshi, N. Hori, T. Recuperative power of a short daytime nap with or without stage 2 sleep. *Sleep.* 2005 Jul 1: 28(7): pp 829-36.

ii) Davidhizar, R. Poole, V. Giger, JN. Power nap rejuvenates body, mind. *Pa Nurse.* 1996 Mar: 51(3): pp 6-7.

iii) Mednick, SC. Nakayama, K. Cantero, JL. Atienza, M. Levin, AA. Pathak, N. Stickgold, R. The restorative benefit of naps on perceptual deterioration. *Nature Neuroscience*, July 2002.

iv) Mednick, SC. Nakayama, K. Stickgold, R. Sleep-dependent learning: A nap is as good as a night. *Nature Neuroscience*, July 2003.

Wisdom Three

1. For more on Don Tolman or his writings on whole food medicine and food signatures, see; Tolman, D. *Farmacist Desk Reference*. 2005. Benaquista Publishing Inc.

2. So, FV. Guthrie, N. et al. Inhibition of human breast cancer cell proliferation and delay of mammary tumorigenesis by flavonoids and citrus juices. *Nutrition & Cancer*, 1996. 26: pp 167-81.

3. Price, WA. *Nutrition and Physical Degeneration*. 1939. Published by Keats Publishing.

4. Ibid. pp 174-79.

5. Thanks to John Robbins for this phrase. *Healthy at 100*. 2006. Random House Publishing. pp 91.

6. i) Willett, WC. et al. Intake of trans fatty acids and risk of coronary heart disease among women. *Lancet*. June 1993: 341. pp 581-585.

    ii) Ascherio, A. et al. Trans-fatty acids intake and risk of myocardial infarction. *Circulation*. 1994: 89. pp 94-101.

7. With thanks to Holly Davis and her great article, 'How much salt is too much'. *Notebook Magazine*. July 2010. pp 68.

    * The quote from Pythagoras also came from this article.

8. From a talk on Self-Care by Don Tolman. June 5, 2010. Shang-ri La Hotel, Sydney.

9. i) Larsson, SC. Orsini, N. Wolk, A. Processed Meat Consumption and Stomach Cancer Risk: A Meta-Analysis; *Journal of the National Cancer Institute* 2006 98(15): pp 1078-1087.

    ii) Cross, AJ. Leitzmann, MF. Gail, MH. Hollenbeck, AR. Schatzkin, A. Sinha, RA. Prospective Study of Red and Processed Meat Intake in Relation to Cancer Risk. *PLoS Med*. 2007: 4(12): e325.

    iii) Larsson, SC. Bergkvist, L. Wolk, A. Processed meat consumption, dietary nitrosamines and stomach cancer risk in a cohort of Swedish women. *Int J Cancer*. 2006 Aug 15;119 (4): pp 915-9.

10. From an independent investigation by The Sun-Herald. See article by Maxine Frith on January 20, 2008—http://www.smh.com.au/news/national/supermarket-apples-10-months-old/2008/01/19/1200620272669.html

11. Tapsell, L. Hemphill, I. Cobiac, L. Sullivan, DR. Fenech, M. Patch, CS. Roodenrys, S. Keogh, JB. Clifton, PM. Williams, PG. Fazio, VA, Inge, KE. Health benefits of herbs and spices: the past, the present, the future. *Medical Journal of Australia.* 2006; 185 (4 Suppl): S1-S24.

12. Dragland, S. Senoo, H. Wake, K. et al. Several culinary and medicinal herbs are important sources of dietary anti-oxidants. J Nutr. 2003. 133: pp 12861290.

13. i) Song et al, Diarylheptanoids with free radical scavenging and hepatoprotective activity in vitro from curcuma longa. 2001. *Plant Med* 67(9). pp 876-877.

    ii) See 12 above.

14. i) Kuttan, P. Potential anticancer activity of turmeric (Curcuma longa). *Cancer Lett.* 1985.Nov:29(2):pp 197-202.

    ii) Miquel, J. Bernd, A. Sempere, JM. Diaz-Alperi, J. and Ramirez, A.(2002). The curcuma anti-oxidants: Pharmacological effects and prospects for future clinical use. A review. *Archives of Gerontology and Geriatrics.* 34.pp 37-46.

    iii) Also see the work of Thomas M. Newmark and Paul Schulick or the book, *The Answer to Cancer* by Dr Hari Sharma MD, Rama K. Mishra and James Meade.pp 43-45.

15. Egan, ME. Pearson, M. Weiner, SA. Rajendran, V. Rubin, D. Glöckner-Pagel, J. Canny, S. Du, K, Lukacs, GL. Caplan MJ. Curcumin, a Major Constituent of Turmeric, Corrects Cystic Fibrosis Defects. *Science.* 23 April 2004: Vol. 304. no. 5670, pp 600—602.

16. Khan, A. Safdar, M. Muzaffar, M. Khan, A. Khattak, KN. Anderson, RA. Cinnamon Improves Glucose and Lipids of People with Type 2 Diabetes. *Diabetes Care.* 2003: 26:pp 3215-3218.

17. Willcox, BJ. Willcox, DC. Suzuki, M. *The Okinawa Program: Learn the Secrets to Health and Longevity.* 2001. Three Rivers Press (Random House).

    For a summary of findings see www.okicent.org.

18. Ibid—particularly the weblink www.okicent.org According to the authors of *The Okinawa Program*, until recently there were approximately 80,000 centenarians in the United States, or about 10—20 centenarians per 100,000 population.* Although regional differences exist, these rates are similar to other developed nations. In Okinawa, centenarian ratios may be the world's highest at approximately 50 per 100,000 population (Japan Ministry of Health, Labor and Welfare, 2006).

   * Precise estimations are difficult since there was no national birth registration system in the US until 1940.

19. Willcox, BJ. Willcox, DC. Suzuki, M. *The Okinawa Program*. 2001. Three Rivers Press (Random House).

20. Bernstein, Willcox et al. JGMS 2004—as reported on www.okicent.org

21. Wilcox, B, Wilcox, DC. and Suzuki, M. *The Okinawa Diet Plan*. 2005. Three Rivers Press (Random House).

22. Caloric Restriction, the Traditional Okinawan Diet, and Healthy Aging: The Diet of the World's Longest-Lived People and Its Potential Impact on Morbidity and Life Span. 2007. *Ann. N.Y. Acad. Sci.* 1114:pp 434–455.

23. Miyagi, S. Iwama, N. Kawabata, T. Hasegawa, K. Longevity and diet in Okinawa, Japan: the past, present and future. *Asia Pac J Public Health.* 2003.15:Suppl:S3-9.

Wisdom Four

1. Leonard, G. '*The Ultimate Athlete*'. 1974. NorThatlantic Books. pp 237-38.

2. Documentary on the Tarahumara Indians—Produced and directed by Marek Maria Baranski. Written by Roy Hanna and Stewart Trotter. Narrated by Rula Lenska. As appeared on the 'People' program. SBS Television. Australia.

3. Ibid.

4. Beare, S. *The Live Longer Diet*, 2003, Piatkus (Little, Brown Book Group).

5. Douillard, J. *Body, Mind and Sport*, 1994. Harmony Books, a division of Random House, Inc.

6. Ramacharaka, Yogi. *The Science of Breath*. © L.N Fowler & Co. Ltd. Cosimo Books. New York.

7.   Leonard, G. *The Ultimate Athlete*. 1974. NorThatlantic Books. pp 160-61.

8.   Ibid. pp 40.

Wisdom Five

1.   i) Pasco, JA. Henry, MJ. Nicholson, GC. et al. Vitamin D status of women in the Geelong Osteoporosis Study: Association with diet and casual exposure to sunlight. *Med J Aust* 2001; 175:pp 401-405.

     ii) McGrath, JJ. Kimlin, MG. Saha, S. et al. Vitamin D insufficiency in southeast Queensland. *Med J Aust* 2001; 174:pp 150-151.

2.   Grover, S. Morley, R. Vitamin D deficiency in veiled or dark-skinned pregnant women. *Med J Aust.* 2001: 175:pp 251-252.

3.   Nowson, C. MacInnis, R. Stein, M. et al. Vitamin D deficiency in residential care facilities in Australia. *Proc Nut Soc Aust.* 2000:pp 24: 154.

4.   Parfitt, AM. Osteomalacia and related disorders. In: Avioli, LV. Krane, SM. eds. Metabolic bone disease and clinically related disorders. 2nd ed. Philadelphia: WB Saunders, 1990:pp 329-96.

5.   Holick, MF. Vitamin D: importance in the prevention of cancers, type 1 diabetes, heart disease, and osteoporosis. *American Journal of Clinical Nutrition*. March 2004. Vol. 79, No. 3.pp 362-371.

6.   Puchacz, E. Stumpf, WE. Stachowiak, EK. Stachowiak, MK. Vitamin D increases expression of the tyrosine hydroxylase gene in adrenal medullary cells. *Brain Res.Mol.* 1996.36:pp 193-6.

7.   Gloth, FM 3rd. Alam, W. Hollis, B. Vitamin D versus broad spectrum phototherapy in the treatment of seasonal affective disorder. *J Nutr Health Aging*. 1999.3(1):pp 5-7.

8.   Holick, MF. Sunlight and vitamin D for bone health and prevention of autoimmune diseases, cancers, and cardiovascular disease. *American Journal of Clinical Nutrition*. December 2004. Vol. 80, No. 6, 1678S-1688S.

9.   Merlino, LA. Curtis, J. Mikuls, TR. Cerhan, JR. Criswell, LA. Saag, KG. Vitamin D intake is inversely associated with rheumatoid arthritis: Results from the Iowa Women's Health Study. *Arthritis and Rheumatism*. 2004.50:1. pp 72-77.

10. Pappa, HM. Gordon, CM. Saslowsky, TM. Zholudev, A. Horr, B. Shih, MC. Grand, RJ. Vitamin D status in children and young adults with inflammatory bowel disease. *Pediatrics* Nov 2006. 118(5).pp 1950—1961.

11. Munger, KL. Zhang, SM. O'Reilly, E. Hernán, MA. Olek, MJ. Willett, WC. Ascherio, A. Vitamin D intake and incidence of multiple sclerosis. *Neurology.* 2004;62:pp 60-65.

12. Munger, KL. Levin, LI. Hollis, BW. Howard, NS. Ascherio, A. Serum 25hydroxyvitamin D levels and risk of multiple sclerosis. *JAMA* 2006; 296:pp 2832-8.

13. Grant, WB. An estimate of premature cancer mortality in the U.S. due to inadequate doses of solar ultraviolet-B radiation. *Cancer.* March 2002; 94: pp 1867-75.

14. Grant, WB. An ecologic study of dietary and solar ultraviolet-B links to breast carcinoma mortality rates. *Cancer* 2002 Jan 1:94 (1):pp 272-81.

15. Lamprecht, SA. Lipkin, M. Cellular mechanisms of calcium and vitamin D in the inhibition of colorectal carcinogenesis. *Ann N Y Acad Sci.* Dec 2001:952:pp 73-87.

16. Mokady, E. Schwartz, B. Shany, S. A protective role of dietary vitamin D3 in rat colon carcinogenesis. *Nutr Cancer.* 2000: 38(1):pp 65-73.

17. Polek, TC. Weigel, NL. Vitamin D and prostate cancer. *J Androl.* 2002 Jan-Feb.23(1):pp 9-17.

18. Tuohimaa, P. Lyakhovich, A. Aksenov, N. Vitamin D and prostate cancer. *J Steroid Biochem Mol Biol.* 2001 Jan-Mar:76(1-5):pp 125-34.

19. i) See Reference 13—Grant, WB.

    ii) Grant, WB. Insufficient Sunlight may kill 45,000 Americans each year from Internal Cancer. *J Col Dermatol.* 2004:3.1:pp 76-78.

    iii) Grant, WB. Garland, CF. Holick, MF. Comparisons of estimated economic burdens due to insufficient solar ultraviolet irradiance and vitamin D and excess solar UV for the United States. *Photochem Photobiol.* 2005. 81: pp 1276-1286.

    iv) Grant, WB. Garland, CF. The association of solar ultraviolet B (UVB) with reducing risk of cancer: multifactorial ecologic analysis of geographic variation in age-adjusted cancer mortality rates. *Anticancer Res.* 2006; 26: pp 2687-99.

20. Godar, DE. Landry, RJ. Lucas, AD. Increased UVA exposures and de-creased cutaneous Vitamin D(3) levels may be responsible for the increas-ing incidence of melanoma. *Med Hypotheses.* 2009 Apr:72(4):pp 434-43.

21. Dr Holick is from the Boston University School of Medicine and is the author of '*The Vitamin D Solution*.'

22. Gilchrest, B. Eller, M. Geller, A. Yaar, M. The Pathogenesis of Melanoma Induced by Ultraviolet Radiation. *The New England Journal of Medicine.* April 29, 1999.

23. See 20. Godar, DE. 2009.

24. This is the recommendation of the Working Group of the Australian and New Zealand Bone and Mineral Society, Endocrine Society of Australia and Osteoporosis Australia.

25. This recommendation comes from the internationally regarded sunlight and vitamin D expert, Krispin Sullivan. For more on her wonderful work, see her book, *Naked at Noon—Understanding Sunlight and Vitamin D.* 2002.

26. Tarran, J. Torpy, F. and Burchett, M. 2007, Use of living pot-plants to cleanse indoor air—research review, Proceedings of 6th International Conf. On In-door Air Quality, Ventilation & Energy Conservation—Sustainable Built Environment, Sendai, Japan, Oct., Vol III.pp 249-256.

27. i) Wood, RA. Burchett, MD. Alquezar, A. Orwell, R. Tarran, J. and Torpy, F. 2006, The potted-plant microcosm substantially reduces indoor air VOC pollution: I. Office field-study, Water, Air, and Soil Pollution: 175.pp 163-180.

    ii) Orwell, R. Wood, R. Burchett, M. Tarran, J. and Torpy, F. 2006, The potted-plant microcosm substantially reduces indoor air VOC pollution: II. Laboratory study, Water, Air, and Soil Pollution:177.pp 59-80.

28. i) Fjeld, T. The effects of plants and artificial daylight on the well-being and health of office workers, school children and health-care personnel, *Proceedings of International Plants for People Symposium*, Floriade, Am-sterdam, NL. 2002. See also,

    ii) Fjeld, T. Veierstebd, LB. Sandvike, L. et al. The effects of foliage plants on health and discomfort symptoms among office workers. 1998. *Indoor Built Environment*, 7: pp 204-209.

Wisdom Six

1. Some of the many journals include The Lancet, International Journal of Neuroscience, Scientific American, American Journal of Cardiology, British Journal of Psychology, Journal of the National Medical Association and Psychosomatic Medicine.

2. Examples of the studies on TM and health include;

Reduced Blood Pressure

Schneider, RH. et al. A randomized controlled trial of stress reduction in the treatment of hypertension in African Americans during one year. *American Journal of Hypertension.* 2005:18(1):pp 88–98.

Reduced Stress

i) Orme-Johnson, DW. and Walton K. W. All approaches of preventing or reversing effects of stress are not the same. *American Journal of Health Promotion.*1998:12:pp 297-299.

ii) Gaylord, C. et al. The effects of the Transcendental Meditation technique and progressive muscle relaxation on EEG coherence, stress reactivity, and mental health in black adults. *International Journal of Neuroscience.* 1989.46:pp 77-86.

Reduced Anxiety

i) Alexander, CN. et al. Effects of the Transcendental Meditation program on stress reduction, health, and employee development: A prospective study in two occupational settings. *Anxiety, Stress and Coping: An International Journal.* 1993. 6:pp 245-262.

ii) Eppley, KR. et al. Differential effects of relaxation techniques on trait anxiety: A meta-analysis. *Journal of Clinical Psychology.* 1989.45:pp 957-974.

Reduced Substance Abuse

Alexander, CN. et al. Treating and preventing alcohol, nicotine, and drug abuse through Transcendental Meditation: A review and statistical metaanalysis. *Alcoholism Treatment Quarterly.* 1994.11:pp 13-87.

Reduced Depression

Ferguson, PC. et al. Psychological Findings on Transcendental Meditation. *Journal of Humanistic Psychology.* 1976.16:pp 483-488.

Increased Brain Function

i) Lyubimov, NN. Electrophysiological characteristics of mobilization of hidden brain reserves. Abstracts, the International Symposium 'Physiological and Biochemical Basis of Brain Activity' (St. Petersburg, Russia: Russian Academy of Science, Institute of the Human Brain).1994:5.

ii) Travis, F. Patterns of EEG coherence, power, and contingent negative variation characterize the integration of transcendental and waking states. *Biological Psychology.* 2002:61:pp 293-319.

Increased Self-Actualization

Alexander, C.N. et al. Transcendental Meditation, self-actualization, and psychological health: A conceptual overview and statistical meta-analysis. *Journal of Social Behavior and Personality*, 1991.6:pp 189–247.

Higher States of Consciousness

Harung, HS. et al. Peak performance and higher states of consciousness: A study of world-class performers. *Journal of Managerial Psychology*, 1996: 11(4):pp 3–23.

3. i) Orme-Johnson, DW. Medical Care Utilization and the Transcendental Meditation Program. *Psychosomatic Medicine.* 1987:49:pp 493-507.

ii) Paul-Labrador, M. Polk, D. Dwyer, JH. Velasquez, I. Nidich, S. Rainforth, M. Schneider, R. Merz, CN. 'Effects of a randomized controlled trial of transcendental meditation on components of the metabolic syndrome in subjects with coronary heart disease'. *Archives of Internal Medicine.* June 2006:166(11):pp 1218–24.

4. Wallace, RK. et al. *International Journal of Neuroscience.*1982:16:pp 53–58.*

* See also,

i) Alexander, CN. et al. Transcendental Meditation, mindfulness, and longevity. *Journal of Personality and Social Psychology.* 1989.57:pp 950-964.

ii) Barnes, VA. et al. Impact of Transcendental Meditation on mortality in older African Americans—eight year follow-up. *Journal of Social Behavior and Personality.* 2005.17(1).pp 201-216.

Wisdom Seven

1. Faith, RE, Murgo, AJ. Plontikoff, NP. Interactions between the immune system and the nervous system. *Stress and immunity*. 1991. CRC, Boca Raton. pp 287-303.

2. Brokensha, G. Clinical intuition: more than rational? *Australian Prescriber*. 2002. Vol 25(1).

3. Thanks to Mia Dalby-Ball for the original input for this exercise.

4. From an essay by Lama Surya Das in Friedman, J. *Earth's Elders—the wisdom of the world's oldest people*. 2005. The quote at the start of the chapter also comes from this essay.

Epilogue

1. Brownstein, A. 'Extraordinary Healing'. Rodale. Originally published by Harbor Press Inc. 2005:pp 206.

Index

THE RAJ

Premier Ayurveda Health Spa

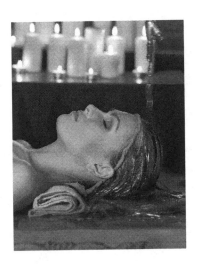

The Raj is one of the world's premier Ayurvedic Health Centers. The only such facility outside of India specifically built to offer the traditional rejuvenation treatments of Ayurveda, it has been featured on Dr.Oz, CBS, NBC, ABC, CNN, and in Time magazine, NY Times, Wall Street Journal, Elle, LA Times, and was listed among *"the best 8 Destination spas."* by Newsweek Magazine.

To give yourself the true gift of Ayurvedic rejuvenation, health and bliss ... from the inside out, check out the wonderful mind-body programs The Raj has to offer.

www.theraj.com

THE DAVID LYNCH FOUNDATION

Combating Traumatic Stress in
At-risk Populations

David Lynch, award-winning US film director established the David Lynch Foundation in 2005.

The foundation funds the implementation of scientifically proven stress-reducing modalities, including the Transcendental Meditation program (TM), for at-risk populations such as underserved inner-city students; veterans with PTSD; female victims of domestic violence; American Indians suffering from diabetes, cardiovascular disease and high suicide rates; homeless men participating in re-entry programs; and incarcerated juveniles and adults.

The aim is to ensure that every child and at-risk adult in the world who wants to learn to meditate can do so.

10% of the profits from this book go to supporting the foundation.

For more information visit
www.davidlynchfoundation.org

ANCIENT WISDOM FOR MODERN HEALTH— 'BOOK TWO'

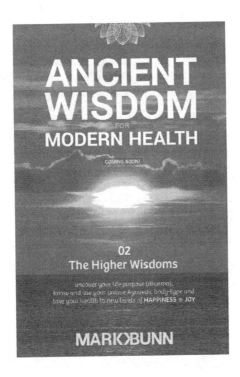

Draft cover only

The second book in Mark Bunn's 'Ancient Wisdom for Modern Health' Series is coming soon. If you liked this book, Book Two—The Higher Wisdoms—will help you take your health to even higher levels.

To Get Notified of When Book TWO is Out ... Go To
markbunn.com.au/book2_notification
or Like Mark's FB Page:
Facebook.com/Mark.Bunn.EasternWisdom

A TASTE OF BOOK TWO—
THE HIGHER WISDOMS

Dharma is the foundation that supports all life
Mahabharata

What if life was as simple as doing one thing? What if doing what we were naturally born to do—our *dharma*—could change our lives from struggle and strain to one of flow, fulfillment and unbounded joy?

Just as no cell in our bodies is without a purpose, the ancient sciences state that each one of us has a certain role in life to fulfill in order to enjoy our highest levels of health and to contribute to the overall health of society. When we find and fulfill out dharma—those activities that support our highest evolution—we spontaneously enjoy our 'natural flow state' and create the state of functioning common to both our highest levels of outer performance as well as the most blissful states of inner contentment.

Whether as a parent, tradesperson, teacher, entertainer, healer, cleaner or support worker, when we use our '*gifts from God*,' as they were known, and perform the jobs or vocations that we were hardwired for, we cultivate the state of *enjoyable ease* that underpins our highest state of health and wellness.

> When we use our innate natural gifts,
> we experience maximum enjoyment.
> When we work for a greater purpose in serving others,
> we experience maximum fulfillment.
> When we combine the two, what greater joy can there be?

To Get Notified of When Book TWO is Out ... Go To
markbunn.com.au/book2_notification
or Like Mark's FB Page:
Facebook.com/Mark.Bunn.EasternWisdom

Like a Motivational Health Speaker for your Conference or Special Event?

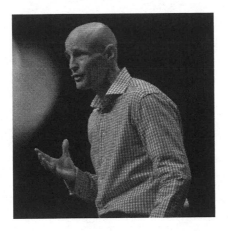

Do you have an upcoming conference or special event and would like to inspire your group to better health and higher performance?

Combining his unique mix of East and West, today Mark Bunn speaks in multiple countries each year entertaining audiences on topics such as natural health, happiness, life balance, Ayurveda, meditation, spirituality and consciousness. His inspiring, uplifting seminars are ideal as a motivating keynote, an energizing workshop, or for simply adding a lighthearted break to a heavy business or association event.

Whether you have an event for business or health professionals, an association or a community-based group, and whether you are in Australia, Asia, the USA or Europe, your audience will love Mark's life-changing talks.

"Mark has a message that delivers an immediate positive impact. He will change the way you think about wellness and quite possibly change your life."
Robert S. Conlee—CEO Neways International—Utah USA
(1400 health-enthusiasts—Adelaide Convention Centre)

MORE INFORMATION

Purchasing More Books & Mark's Free Newsletters

To purchase <u>further copies of this book (or the ebook or audio CD versions of the book)</u>, visit www.markbunn.com.au/products

To receive <u>a free subscription to Mark's 'Ancient Wisdom for Modern Health' online newsletter</u>, go to www.markbunn.com.au/etips

Spreading the Word

Mark's fundamental passion and purpose in writing this book has been to remind people that staying healthy and well is not as complicated or confusing as we have been led to believe. It is his heartfelt wish that individually and collectively, more of us can re-embrace the simple wisdoms of health and happiness.

If you enjoyed this book, we would love you to help spread the word by letting as many other people as possible know about it (Facebook, Twitter, email, blogs, newsletters etc). If we can help you do this in any way, just let us know at info@markbunn.com.au

Alternatively, simply send a personal recommendation to friends, associates, groups you are involved in, with a link to

www.markbunn.com.au/products

Connect with Mark

markbunn.com.au

(Author page): facebook.com/Mark.Bunn.EasternWisdom

(Personal): facebook.com/markbunn.ancientwisdom

linkedin.com/in/markbunn

twitter.com/mark_bunn

youtube.com/user/MarkBunn

info@markbunn.com.au

Made in the USA
San Bernardino, CA
12 February 2019